THE
Amino
REVOLUTION

ROBERT ERDMANN, Ph.D.
with Meirion Jones

A FIRESIDE BOOK
Published by Simon & Schuster
New York   London   Toronto   Sydney   Tokyo

F

Fireside
Simon & Schuster Building
Rockefeller Center
1230 Avenue of the Americas
New York, New York 10020

Copyright © 1987 by Robert Erdmann and Meirion Jones

First Fireside Edition, 1989
Published by arrangement with Contemporary Books
FIRESIDE and colophon are registered trademarks
of Simon & Schuster Inc.
Manufactured in the United States of America

9   10   8   Pbk.

Library of Congress Cataloging-in-Publication Data
Erdmann, Robert.
The amino revolution/Robert Erdmann with Meirion Jones.—
1st Fireside ed.
p.   cm.
Reprint. Originally published: Chicago: Contemporary Books, c1987.
"A Fireside book."
Bibliography: p.
1. Amino acids in human nutrition.   2. Amino acids—
Therapeutic use.   3. Dietary supplements.   I. Jones, Meirion.
II. Title.
[QP561.E73   1989]
613.2′8—dc19   89-4321
CIP
ISBN 0-671-67359-9

To globs of amino acids in the form of future generations, to patients, and to lovers all over the world. May they enjoy the best of health. R.E.

To Mark Matschler and Jackie Ayers. M.J.

Contents

Authors' Note

The authors of this book have developed this program to inform the reader of new options in the field of nutritional supplementation. This information is for educational purposes only, and is not meant to take the place of the advice of a qualified health care professional.

Although in clinical practice amino acids have been used safely *as outlined in this book*, it is important that you consult with your doctor before you undertake this or any new health regimen. If, after you have added one or more nutritional supplements, a condition appears, persists, or worsens, stop taking the supplement immediately, and call a physician.

Warning: Phenylketonurics (those suffering from PKU), anyone on a phenylalanine-restricted diet, patients being treated for high blood pressure, schizophrenics, and those taking MAO inhibitor drugs (antidepressants), should carefully read Chapter 5, "Safety and Precautions," and should not embark upon a program of amino acid supplementation without a doctor's consent and monitoring. And as with any health program, pregnant women and parents of young children should discuss nutritional changes of *any sort* with an appropriate health care professional before making them.

Foreword

It so often happens that our vision of search is toward the horizon, little realizing that what we are seeking lies at our own feet. We look for remedies in drugs while completely overlooking the body's need for missing nutritional links. The *cause* of malfunction is deficiency, whereas the *effect* of the malfunction may be disease. In such an instance, the true method of treatment is to rectify the cause, and not to quell the effect with drugs and leave the cause untreated.

Amino acids work as bodybuilding blocks, protectors of the cells, alleviators of pain, generators of ecstasy, and guardians of health. In fact the whole process of well-being depends upon them. They can shield us from the modern world's menaces of radiation and pollution, and can definitely present a way to combat the aging process. Free amino acids can also help against allergies and autoimmune diseases.

When I was seeking an antiaging program for my clinic, I turned to Dr. Robert Erdmann; he is a brilliant nutritionist, and completely dedicated to his profession. He produces near-miraculous results in patients and infuses a degree of well-being they claim never to have enjoyed before. His answer to rejuvenation in humans does not lie in the "monkey gland" or placental extracts, but in the synergistic action of free amino acids, vitamins, and minerals.

This book tells you how to increase the efficiency of your body. It is a guiding light that some will follow and some ignore; such is the nature of things. It is my pleasure to recommend it as an invaluable guide to well-being.

D. Basra, M.D.
Fellow of the Royal College of Surgeons

As the twentieth century draws to a close, we are entering a Golden Age of medicine, in which the traditional medical boundaries are rapidly changing and we are beginning to focus on the causes of illness and ways to help the body heal itself. More and more, we are realizing that the physical body is a complex biochemical machine. Nutritional medicine is the new frontier in medicine and is dedicated to the nontoxic, natural, and safe care of our biochemical selves.

It is generally accepted that the body needs adequate amounts of certain vitamins and minerals in order to be "healthy." Amino acids are important, but often neglected, components of the magical balance we call health. Amino acids, often called the "building blocks of protein," make up a large portion of the human body, including muscle and connective tissue, and play a vital role in maintaining the biochemical balance that gives us energy and helps our organs function smoothly. In *The Amino Revolution*, Dr. Erdmann simplifies and clarifies the complex concepts of amino acid biochemistry, making correct amino acid supplementation a possibility for all those interested in health and nutrition.

Dr. Erdmann has helped me expand my knowledge of practical nutritional and preventive medical care by sharing his considerable expertise in the new field of amino supplementation. In *The Amino Revolution*, Dr. Erdmann offers *everyone* interested in better health a thoughtful, clinically relevant, timely insight into the complex world of amino acids. With this book, Dr. Erdmann enables all individuals seeking a greater understanding of nutrition and health to better take care of one of the most marvelous creations on earth—the human body.

Carol A. Shamlin, M.D.

This remarkable book speaks about the use of free-form amino acids as part of a total self-care approach to metabolic nutrition where vitamins, minerals, and other natural substances are used to rectify whatever biochemical imbalances prevent someone from living at a high level of vitality and well-being. It is an approach which makes it possible not only to help an ailing body to heal itself but, even more important, to keep a well one well and to protect it from premature aging and degenerative illness.

I first came upon some of the near-miracles which free-form amino acids could perform ten years ago when I met forward-thinking doctors in the United States using them to treat ailments as diverse as manic-depression, anxiety, poor memory, high blood pressure, sexual problems, and arthritis. Ever since, I have wanted to see someone truly knowledgeable about their use, produce a guide for the general public. *The Amino Revolution* is such a guide— and responsibly so for it never advocates the use of these potent building blocks of nature without full nutritional support from the cofactor vitamins and minerals necessary to make efficient and safe use of them as part of a total nutritional program.

To stay alive and healthy the body continuously uses energy. This energy, which has its ultimate origins in the sun, is made available to us thanks to the special biochemical transformations which we as living creatures are able to perform. In a young and healthy body these transformations are carried out in miraculously ordered ways thanks to a supply of raw materials—vitamins, minerals, amino acids, essential fatty acids, and other metabolites—being available in abundance. Interwoven, interacting, and interdependent in highly elaborate ways, these biochemical transformations make the world's most advanced computer look like a child's toy. Each takes place in a series of chemical steps. These chemical chains of events which begin with a single molecule and proceed by changing one thing into another until your body has made the specific substance it needs for a particular purpose are known as metabolic pathways—the means by which all life processes are carried out. And the healthy human body is a biological masterpiece with superbly balanced mechanisms. Erdmann and Jones understand well that high-level health depends entirely upon maintaining such a dynamic biochemical balance. When something goes wrong with the balance—either as a result of stress, or poor diet, or microbial invasion—then illness ensues. Just what kind of illness and just how serious depends upon your inherited weaknesses and on the strength of your immune system.

The Erdmann-Jones metabolic approach to nutrition attempts to supply your body with what it needs to maintain its own health or to heal itself from within. This it does by making sure that as many as possible of the body's highly complex metabolic pathways have the specific nutrients they require in optimal amounts to function smoothly and efficiently.

Their book is based on an extremely simple yet profound nuts-and-bolts hypothesis which goes something like this: our bodies are quite literally constructed out of vitamins, minerals, amino acids, fatty acids, and other metabolites derived from them, working together according to a living molecular logic. Because we are alive, that life provides us with the consciousness to utilize these nuts and bolts via this elaborate network of superbly engineered and interlocking metabolic pathways. So, if we can discover exactly which nuts and bolts in the form of vitamins and minerals, amino acids, and essential fatty acids are needed in extraordinary amounts, or are simply in short supply in our bodies, and then to be able to increase those amounts, all will be well.

Erdmann himself is an extraordinary combination of in-depth knowledge and highly developed intuition and inventiveness. His coauthor Meirion Jones is a young man of exceptional intelligence with the ability to put into simple and often highly amusing language even the most complex information. Together, I believe they have written a book which will be of enormous help to anyone, well or unwell, who has asked the question "How can I look and feel better than I do right now?"

Leslie Kenton,
health expert and author of
Ageless Aging and *The Biogenic Diet*

Preface

My interest in nutrition, and its importance in health care, was sparked by my mother. I remember as a child hearing her say that good nutrition was vital for our well-being. She made the whole family take cod liver oil and would often sprinkle wheat germ on our food. Even so, at that time there was so little awareness of the dangers of refined foods that, along with every other child in the neighborhood, no sooner was I out of the house than I was stuffing my face with sweets.

Years later, following my qualification as a psychologist, I found myself drawn to the way that behavior was influenced by food. I knew that simple things such as hunger could cause loss of concentration and irritability, but what really fascinated me were tests showing how vitamin C supplements could actually raise the IQs of schoolchildren. Conversely a shortage of important nutrients was found to lower IQ and lead to general underachievement.

It seemed obvious that, as my mother had insisted, good nutrition was essential for both physical and mental health. Yet when I tried to discuss this with my brother, a medical doctor, he told me that his entire training in nutrition had consisted of a single morning lecture. Realizing how undervalued the notion of good nutrition is in health care, but convinced of its importance, I decided to find out everything I could about the subject. I felt that the best way to learn was to devise and teach a course in "Superhealth." My idea was that, rather than treating people's illnesses, I would give healthy people the nutritional information they needed to stay healthy. My plan was to help them avoid getting ill in the first place.

As I became more deeply involved in this idea, discovering all I could about the application of nutritional supplements, I came across the largely unexplored area of amino acid therapy. I quickly recognized the importance of amino acids in maintaining the vitality of mind and body. It changed the direction of my clinical practice. Since then, my understanding of the workings of the body has grown rapidly.

The benefits of taking supplements of amino acids to improve your health can hardly be overstated. All the body's tissue—every cell, muscle, hair, nail, enzyme, and brain chemical—is made from amino acids. They are central to the biochemistry of your body.

I use amino acid supplements, together with the vitamins and minerals the body needs to help metabolize them, in my nutritional counseling practice. I have come to believe that most illnesses, even viral and bacterial ones, result from nutritional deficiencies. The essence of my practice lies in discovering which substances are missing or in short supply, then providing them to the patient as supplements. With this philosophy—using nutritional supplementation—I have helped the victims of a wide variety of psychological complaints and physical disorders. Furthermore, giving patients the nutrition they need to make them healthy shifts the focus from sickness to health, and to what it takes to stay healthy.

This book sets out to explain my working methods, examining the theory behind nutritional counseling as well as looking at its success in practice. You'll see how different illnesses and disorders respond to different combinations of high-potency amino acid supplements. I am convinced that this form of therapy, which includes vitamin and mineral cofactors, offers great hope for health care in the future. And I hope that, after reading the book, you'll agree.

Robert Erdmann

Acknowledgments

L. Kenton, X. Williams, A. Kalokerinos, G. Dettman, M. Burke, R. Cathcart III, W. Belfield, W. Shock, L. Shock, P. Emau, G. Jones, M. Erdmann, C. Shamlin, L. Rose, R. Kunin, M. Lessor, B. Belag, A. Levine, J. Patrick, I. Stone, G. Gordon.

THE
Amino
REVOLUTION

Introduction

Is it possible to ease pain, soothe anxiety, and improve sexual performance simply by taking dietary supplements? If these supplements happen to be free-form amino acids, then the answer is yes. Quite simply, the widespread introduction of amino acids in the form of powders, pills, or capsules is the most exciting advance in health and nutrition in 25 years. The aim of this book is to show you why. In the following pages, you'll see how amino acids can be used to improve both mental and physical vitality, reduce body fat, relieve emotional disorders, and even combat viral infections.

AMINOS, NUTRITION, AND FOOD

Amino acids aren't a new medical discovery. In fact, in their natural state they form the basis of life itself. They are the essential raw materials in the growth or reproduction of every cell of your body. Selected aminos are present in your enzymes and immune system. Every bone, organ, and muscle and almost all hormones are made from combinations of aminos, often with the help of vitamins and minerals. Aminos are metabolic building blocks—without them there would be no life.

Until recently, most doctors believed that taking supplements of pure, or "free form," amino acids as a means of improving health was unnecessary. After all, they reasoned, protein is only a combination of amino acids in the form of long molecular chains, and as most diets are so abundant in protein, it's likely that we can get all the amino acids we need simply from the food we eat. Admittedly, in a perfect world this would be true. Unfortunately, in the real world countless factors are working to prevent our bodies from receiving a full and balanced supply of these all-important substances. Among these factors are the pollution caused by burning fossil fuels, the hormones fed to cattle, the intensive use of fertilizers in agriculture, and even habits such as smoking and drinking, all of which can prevent our bodies from fully using what we eat.

Worse still is the amount of nutrition that is lost from our food through processing before we actually get to eat it. A famous experiment into the effects of food processing was conducted by Professor Francis Pottenger. Taking two groups of kittens, he fed one group on fresh meat, the other on an exclusive diet of canned (processed) cat food. In time, the kittens in both groups grew to maturity and produced litters of their own. With each succeeding generation, the cats fed on fresh food flourished—their fur was glossy and sleek, their behavior lively and alert. The cats in the canned-food group, on the other hand, suffered a gradual physical and mental deterioration—growth was stunted, they became increasingly psychotic and unsociable, and eventually they were unable to reproduce.

Of course, our diets are much more varied than those used in this controlled experiment—we eat a diversity of meat, dairy products, and vegetables. Nevertheless, Pottenger's experiment suggests that no matter how nutritious or tasty our food seems, we still may not be receiving everything we need for a healthy, balanced lifestyle. For confirmation of this point you need only look at the rise in the incidence of disorders such as cancer, heart disease, nervous breakdowns, and anxiety neuroses. This is where free-form amino acid supplements come in. By providing the body with optimal nutrition, amino acids help to replace what is lost and, in doing so, promote well-being and vitality.

A FRESH LOOK AT HEALTH

As you read through the book, you'll realize that an important key to using amino acids is possessing a clear understanding of what health really means. By the standards of conventional medicine, it is defined as the absence of disease—when there are no identifiable symptoms of illness, the patient is said to be well. By the same token, when an illness does occur, it is often treated as an isolated phenomenon that has arisen independent of the rest of the body. In these cases, drugs are prescribed to suppress the symptoms, often with no thought of the deeper and longer-term consequences.

On the other hand, using amino acids means adopting a radically different attitude. It means considering the inner workings of your body, where the reactions of each individual substance cause reactions elsewhere. These reactions are called metabolic pathways. You will be reading a lot about them in this book.

Metabolic pathways are the body's biochemical assembly lines, which take the raw materials, such as the newly eaten amino acids, and manufacture finished products to help the body to live. These finished products include everything from enzymes for digestion to mineral and amino chains for bones and teeth. Making certain that the metabolic pathways work at peak performance—that they meet your body's precise molecular demands—means ensuring that your body has all the raw materials it needs: vitamins, minerals, and, most important of all, amino acids.

A REVOLUTION IN HEALTH

So what can amino acids offer that conventional medicine can't? Can they be used as an AIDS vaccine? In brain scans? No, in both cases. Instead, amino acids are demonstrating an equally valuable lesson. They are making us aware of our bodies as the supremely harmonious organisms that they are. We are beginning to see how every illness, each faltering loss of vitality and well-being, is the result of metabolic imbalances, rather than a single specific cause.

These imbalances can be rectified with nutritional supplementation. In other words, with extra supplements of the raw materials found in the food we eat every day of our lives—that is, amino acids, together with certain vitamins and minerals—we can enhance our health and vitality as never before.

In *The Amino Revolution*, you'll see what this means in practice. By examining the metabolic imbalances behind a variety of health problems, you'll find out which aminos are involved. Then, suggestions for specific combinations of individual free-form aminos show how to restore balance to the affected pathway. In this way, you can strengthen your immune system against infection and disease, restore emotional and mental balance, overcome the bad habits of a lifetime (such as smoking), and generally create enormous vitality—enough to meet the immense demands of the twentieth century.

If you are used to thinking of improving your health by taking single nutritional supplements—such as vitamin C for a cold, or worse, drugs that only suppress the cold's symptoms—this new amino-based approach could radically alter your attitude and expectations. Used wisely, amino acid supplements are miracles of nature. They are safe, simple, and unequaled among natural substances for their health-enhancing potential. The title of this book is no exaggeration. Thanks to amino acids, we are poised at the edge of a revolution in health.

PART ONE
MEET THE FREE AMINOS

1

The Amino Acid
Impact

The 24-hour endurance race at the Spa circuit in Belgium is second only to Le Mans for the demands it makes on competitors. Although each member of a team of three drivers takes turns at driving their car, the race is a grueling test of will and strength. During the July 1986 race, this was especially true for one driver, Allan Moffat. With a teammate overcome by heat exhaustion halfway through the race, Moffat was forced to drive two shifts in a row. The stifling heat, the cabin reverberating with engine noise, the almost superhuman level of concentration, and the continuous gear changes demanded more from him than anyone had a right to expect. Yet, thanks in large part to Moffat's driving, his team received many of the after-race trophies, including the prestigious Kings' Cup.

The most remarkable thing about this race is that, only a matter of days before, Moffat himself had been ill, the victim of a debilitating, six-week-long virus infection. During this period, he had endured such a bad headache that at times he said he thought his eyes "would force their way out of my head." On top of this, he was constantly tired and felt his strength fading day by day. Antibiotics had done nothing but make him sleepy, and as the day of the race approached, he feared that he would have to drop out for the good of the team.

Then, with only a few days to go, Moffat came to me for nutritional counseling. Explaining his symptoms and the contest ahead, he asked if anything could be done at such short notice to prepare him physically for the race. I immediately suggested a high-potency nutritional formula that included vitamins and minerals. The single most important part of this blend, though, was a selection of certain amino acid supplements. These aminos were especially chosen to boost Moffat's energy levels, giving him the vitality to withstand the stresses of the race and to stave off the effects of the virus. They worked so well that, in addition to covering for his codriver, Moffat was the only member of his team with enough strength left to collect their trophies. As his wife said later, "I'd never seen him look so good after a race in all the years I've known him."

Moffat's case isn't an isolated one. More and more people are finding that supplementing their diets with amino acids is one of the most effective and thorough ways of ensuring their health and vitality. Free-form amino acids (that is, amino acids that have been separated in the laboratory from their parent protein molecules) are being hailed as one of this century's greatest advances in medical care.

In later chapters—quoting up-to-the-minute research and the case histories of many people whose physical and mental illnesses have been relieved by amino acids—we'll show you how to use these remarkable substances. Whether you suffer from mood disorders such as depression and anxiety, illnesses such as peptic ulcers, virus infections, or heart problems, whether you have difficulty losing weight, find it impossible to stop smoking or drinking, or simply have a sievelike memory, amino acids can help you.

But before all this, let's find out exactly what amino acids are. How do they work in the body? Why is amino acid supplementation so effective? As amino acids are involved in almost every body function, answering these questions means exploring the way your skin and bones are formed, how organs function, and what enables you to grow, heal, and resist disease.

THE METABOLIC REPUBLIC

Your body is an incredibly complex organism. Imagine it for a moment as a massive, self-contained city. It really isn't such a fanciful comparison. Your cells, after all, are a teeming population of many races and occupations. The arteries are a network of main roads used constantly by high-speed couriers, taxis, semis, and garbage trucks. As in any city, there is a vast and varied communications network. The city has factories, supermarkets, power stations, and beautifully designed architectural wonders; it can even boast its own civil-defense militia.

However, this comparison has one flaw: Cities are randomly gathered groupings of people and institutions, each working for its own separate interests. Everything in your body, on the other hand, exists and works solely for one purpose—to keep you alive and healthy. And proteins—or, more specifically, amino acids—play an incredibly important role in this process.

THE NUTRIENTS OF LIFE

Your food comes in three basic forms: carbohydrates, fats, and proteins. The first two are simply structured. Carbohydrate, for example, exists only as a few variations of glucose and fructose, and most of what you need of these can be made in the body itself. Fats are almost as simple. They take the form of lecithin or cholesterol, or as three fat molecules combined, called triglycerides. The third food, protein, is very different.

The word *protein* is Greek and means "first things." While there are only three or four forms each of fat and carbohydrate in the human body, there are at least fifty thousand recognized forms of protein. This enormous number of differing protein structures gives your body its versatility. All enzymes and most hormones, every cell and muscle, and every piece of tissue from blood vessel to eyeball are made of protein. Three-quarters of all the solid matter in your body is protein. Without it, we would have no teeth and bones, no nervous system, no life.

Each of the fifty thousand proteins in your body must be custom-built to specifications that are peculiar to your body and to no one else's; simply reusing the protein you eat would never meet these specifications. To give you an idea why, imagine an architect dismantling Stonehenge in order to build an ornate mansion from the stone. Obviously, it would be impossible to use the massive granite slabs as they are. So before the builders can go to work, the slabs have to be broken apart and chiseled into various shapes to form keystones, sills, and fluting. Only when this process is finished can the segments of rock be reconstructed to make the house. In the same way, the protein you eat is broken up into smaller constituents and then reconstructed in a different form to meet your body's exact needs. These tiny constituent parts, the building blocks of your body, are amino acids.

When your body needs a particular protein, the amino acids required to make it are bonded together into chains called peptides. These chains of amino acids then combine to form a protein molecule. Protein molecules may contain thousands of amino acids—many of which are the same type, but bonded in specific sequences. Each time another amino acid is added, the chain becomes a new and separate protein with different properties and different functions in the body. This is what enables one chain to become a digestive enzyme and another, with a different sequence of amino acids, a molecule of muscle tissue. It also explains how the approximately twenty amino acids can form at least fifty thousand separate protein structures.

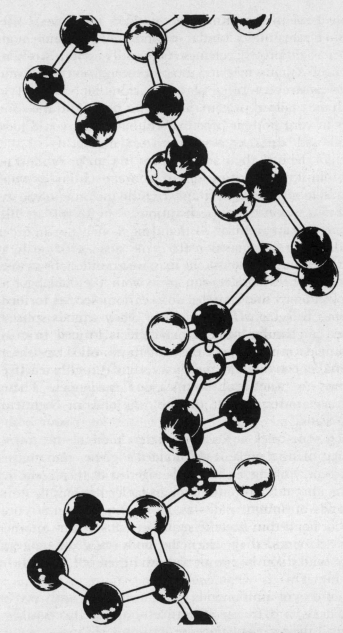

Model of a collagen (fibrous protein) helix. The spheres represent the individual constituents of the amino acids, linked into the orderly, repeating pattern of the collagen molecule.

These protein structures are divided into two basic groups—fibrous and globular proteins. As its name suggests, fibrous protein creates essentially solid, straight tissue, such as muscle. With the single exception of fibroin (a relatively simple form of fibrous protein that creates silk), all fibrous proteins are helix-shaped. This is a versatile shape that allows many protein strands to splice together and increases the overall strength and flexibility of the molecule. Helix-shaped fibrous proteins make up everything from skin tissue to tendons, from muscle and organs to glands, blood vessels, and nerve endings. Even bones are made from a latticework of amino-based protein, with calcium phosphate filling in the gaps.

To perform their tasks (such as flexing or dilating), fibrous proteins must respond to specific orders from the brain. It is the second group of proteins—globular proteins—that carry these orders. Unlike the molecules formed by fibrous protein, which consist of many strands spliced together, a globular protein molecule is formed from a long, single, uninterrupted protein strand rolled up like a ball of wool. It is this that makes the soluble, highly reactive chemicals we know as enzymes and hormones. These substances are responsible for the thousands of chemical reactions that take place every second to keep your body alive. Enzymes pick up two or more chemicals the body needs and bring them together to create a new substance— for example, linking amino acids together to form muscle. The way that this new substance is formed from others is known as a metabolic pathway. Hormones are the driving force behind all your body's metabolic pathways: by activating the enzymes, they order the body to grow, trigger puberty, make you happy or sad, and even tell you when you're hungry.

The ability of amino acids to create either highly active chemicals or hard, fibrous structures shows their versatility. But for all their variety, they are still only chains—minute molecular strands. How do these tiny chains form the complex and robust structures of your body? Picture a beautifully trimmed hedge, surrounding a lawn on three sides. It is so well tended that it looks like one continuous plant—almost a solid wall. In fact, we know it is made up of many smaller plants whose branches have become closely intertwined. The same holds true for protein molecules. By cross-linking and intertwining with other molecule chains of the same protein, they form multilayered latticeworks. Then, folding back on themselves, forming loops and superimposing themselves on other latticeworks, they gradually build up into the highly complicated and specialized three-dimensional structures that make up everything in your body, from teeth to nerve fibers.

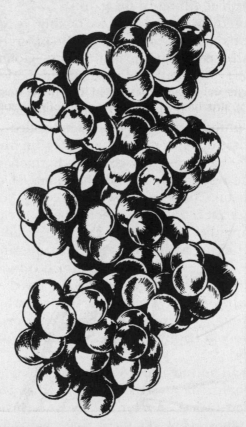

Three collagen strands are wound around each other, creating a resilient and tensile collagen cable.

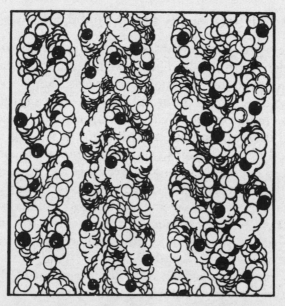

Many collagen cables are cross-linked to form the tough, fibrous "scaffolding" structures of the body's connective tissue.

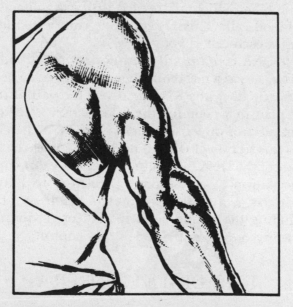

Connective tissue constitutes the bulk of our skin, muscles, and organs, as well as a large part of the structure of our bones.

BLUEPRINTS OF METABOLISM

Imagine a group of newly digested aminos ready to be used somewhere in the body. They have been digested but are as yet unchanged by metabolic pathways. Since every cell manufactures several thousand new proteins a minute, even a minor change in the way that the aminos are linked could result in illness or mutation. Although the job of enzymes is to link different aminos, and of hormones to order any process to begin, they could never meet the huge demands themselves. Instead two substances exist solely for this purpose—deoxyribonucleic acid (DNA) and ribonucleic acid (RNA). These two nucleic acids, widely distributed in human tissue, play a major role in heredity as well as in protein synthesis.

DNA can be looked upon as the blueprint of the entire body. Every piece of information on the way the body is built is encoded in its strands. One part might tell you which aminos and enzymes are needed for a piece of skin tissue, another which are needed in the manufacture of a white blood cell. This genetic code can be found in the nucleus of each cell of your body.

While DNA contains all the information of body structure, RNA acts as a metabolic index. If your body needs, say, some muscle fiber, the RNA discovers the part of the DNA master plan that contains the information needed for the relevant piece of protein synthesis. The RNA then attaches itself to this section of DNA. The RNA assumes the shape of this part of the DNA, becoming in fact an exact copy. This copy is known as a ribosome. Detaching itself from the DNA, it acts as a pattern for protein synthesis, attracting and binding the amino acids in the correct number and sequence according to the code it has copied.

THE DIGESTION TRAP

The protein synthesis just described takes place continuously almost everywhere in the body. It seems to be such a precise operation—the different substances all reacting together in harmony—that it might easily lull you into thinking that nothing could possibly go awry. But you'd be wrong. The very fact that your body is such a delicate and exact mechanism leaves it vulnerable. Even if something seemingly minor goes wrong, you can become prone to illness and disorder.

Imagine, for example, that you have a toothache, and it forces you to swallow your food without chewing it properly. Normally, chewing tears your food apart, enabling the digestive juices to attack a large surface area. The more thoroughly you chew, the greater the amount of nutrients your body will absorb. On the other hand, inadequate chewing leaves a smaller surface area of the food available for the acids and enzymes to work on; when it reaches the small intestine, less of it is digested. This means fewer amino acids are absorbed into the body to continue the vital protein synthesis. As one of the important roles of protein synthesis is to manufacture digestive enzymes, your toothache will be indirectly responsible for the production of fewer enzymes to digest your food. This enzyme depletion worsens the problems created by inadequate chewing and fewer amino acids are released from the food, further depleting the enzyme supply.

Of course, your digestive tract won't be the only thing to suffer. As we've seen, different combinations of amino acids are needed to perform different functions in the body. As these aminos become depleted, their functions are carried out inadequately. Sooner or later, hormone production will drop; there will be less insulin to regulate your blood sugar levels, less adrenalin to help you cope with stress, less thyroxin to carry out body metabolism, and less thymosin to stimulate your immune system. As supplies of the aminos that form fibrous proteins are reduced, your nails will get softer and start to split, your skin will lose its pliability, and muscle tone will fade. Fats, which depend on proteins to be mobilized, will start to build up in your blood vessels, leading to higher blood pressure. You will get tired easily, find everyday situations stressful, and suffer from periods of anxiety and depression. You will become much more susceptible to disease. You will age prematurely. At best, the quality of your life will be much lower than it should be. At worst, you will die.

This picture—suggesting that you can suffer from mental and physical illness simply from one painful molar—might seem a bit extreme. It is, but not by much. It shows how dependent the body is on a balanced supply of amino acids, and how easily an imbalance can be caused, affecting areas of the body that would seem to have no connection at all with your toothache. And there are many things besides bad teeth that can lead to this digestive imbalance. You could make a long list of factors that include emotional stress, junk food, inadequate exercise, viruses, pollution, injury, drug taking (marijuana plays havoc with the secretion of stomach acid), and genetic disorders that affect protein synthesis. They will all decrease the output of digestive chemicals, and so reduce the availability of amino acids that are needed to maintain normal body functions. In time, this nutritional deficiency will allow health disorders to take hold throughout the body, and they can set in motion a destructive chain that will quickly spiral out of control. The way that nutritional deficiencies affect the body resembles one of those spectacular attempts to set a new domino-toppling record. The organizers arrange the dominoes in a pattern with many rows radiating out from the starting point. When the first domino is pushed over, it causes several rows to topple at once, until dominoes are falling simultaneously all around the room. The same holds true of the body's metabolic pathways. A single minor deficiency can easily affect the whole body, unbalancing the entire metabolic network and causing illness.

This is where amino acid supplements come in. We've seen how important these building blocks of protein are to the body. We'll look at which foods contain which aminos in Chapter 3. However, rather than having to depend simply on the protein you get from the food you eat to protect you from illness, you can now add amino supplements to your diet, choosing from powders, capsules, or tablets. They contain nothing but pure individual amino acids. By learning how each disorder affects the different metabolic pathways of your body, you can relieve the disorder by using free-form amino acids to replenish and support the pathways. Thanks to this free-form approach, none of us need ever suffer a shortage of any vital substance. If, for example, you wanted to cure the digestive trouble started by your bad tooth, you could take a supplement containing a blend of the amino acids your body uses to make its digestive enzymes. In its free-form state, this blend is absorbed straight into the body, regardless of digestive difficulties. In this case, your pancreas can use it to manufacture all the enzymes needed to digest your food properly.

With the relevant blends of aminos, this method is equally effective for mood disorders, skin complaints, virus infections, heart disease, premature aging, and cravings for alcohol and cigarettes. All these problems, after all, result from metabolic pathways having been disrupted by nutritional deficiencies. The key to relieving these disorders is to discover which amino deficiencies are responsible for which disorder. Then, by adding supplements of those aminos to your diet—together with the important vitamin and mineral cofactors (which the body often needs to help the conversion process of the metabolic pathways)—you can cure it. This is the theory that lies at the heart of free-form amino acid therapy.

Amino acids aren't drugs. They won't suppress the symptoms of your illness while avoiding the causes. These remarkable powders work solely by strengthening the natural metabolic reactions in your body that allow you to live. Such reactions—the metabolic pathways—are an integral part of amino acid therapy, so understanding how they work is very important.

2

How Aminos Work

Metabolic pathways are like maps. They chart the directions that amino acids, vitamins, and minerals take in the body once they are digested, indicating which substances are needed for which transformations. Using metabolic pathways, the body can choose to employ the same type of amino acid molecule in many different roles. For example, the amino acid might join an RNA pattern and become part of a fibrous protein molecule. Or it may undergo several transformation stages—reacting with various enzymes, minerals, and vitamins—to become another amino with very different properties from the first; perhaps only then will this molecule be used in an RNA pattern. Then again, it may end up as a hormone or as part of an enzyme, which will itself be used to effect transformations on other aminos. The accompanying chart shows the general metabolic pathways in the body.

How the amino acid is used, and which metabolic pathway is chosen, ultimately depends on your body's needs at that moment. If your body needs digestive enzymes, for example, then by transforming the relevant amino acids, your metabolic pathways will supply them. The same goes for connective tissue, hormones, blood vessels, hair, teeth, and antibodies—indeed, for every structure in your body.

METABOLIC PATHWAYS AT WORK

To see how this works in practice, let's examine the different metabolic pathways affecting one of the body's most important amino acids: tryptophan. First, as with most aminos, some of the freshly digested tryptophan molecules immediately join an RNA pattern to assist in creating structural protein such as skin and muscle. Others are used in the formation of bone marrow, which is crucial to the immune system.

Once these needs are satisfied, most of the remaining tryptophan molecules are transformed by two chemical reactions into a hormone called serotonin. Serotonin is an inhibitory neurotransmitter, a brain chemical that is responsible for sending us to sleep at night, relaxing us during the day, preventing us from overreacting to stress, and guarding against uncontrolled rises in blood pressure. To convert to serotonin, tryptophan must first react with the vitamins B_6 and C. Unfortunately, these two vitamins are vulnerable to environmental hazards and can actually be destroyed by cigarette smoke and alcohol. Without them, the tryptophan-serotonin pathway becomes blocked, and there simply is too little serotonin produced to meet your needs. The immediate results of this deficiency are insomnia, increasing tension, and anxiety. In the longer term, serotonin deficiency can lead to chronic depression and a possible rise in blood pressure.

These symptoms alone are enough to suggest that the serotonin-producing metabolic pathway is blocked. However, nutritionists can also detect the problem from a rise in the urinary levels of xanthurenic acid (a form of tryptophan), for with nothing else to do with tryptophan, the body literally pours it away. From these clues, nutritionists can deduce that a patient is suffering from a deficiency of

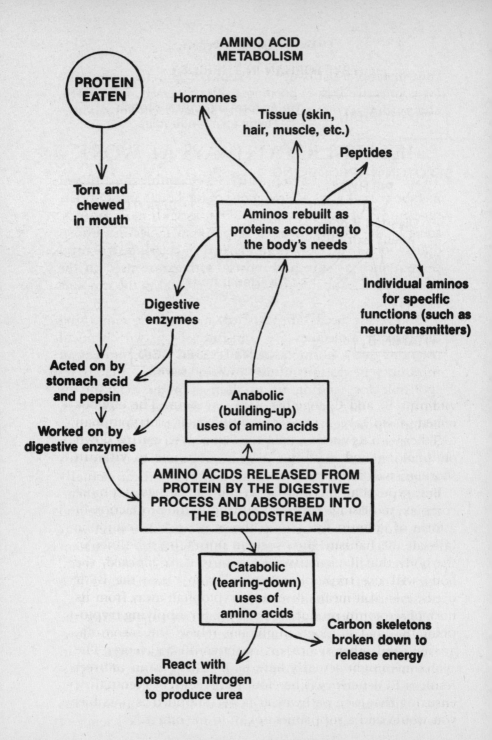

AMINO ACID METABOLISM

PROTEIN EATEN

Hormones

Tissue (skin, hair, muscle, etc.)

Peptides

Torn and chewed in mouth

Aminos rebuilt as proteins according to the body's needs

Digestive enzymes

Individual aminos for specific functions (such as neurotransmitters)

Acted on by stomach acid and pepsin

Anabolic (building-up) uses of amino acids

Worked on by digestive enzymes

AMINO ACIDS RELEASED FROM PROTEIN BY THE DIGESTIVE PROCESS AND ABSORBED INTO THE BLOODSTREAM

Catabolic (tearing-down) uses of amino acids

Carbon skeletons broken down to release energy

React with poisonous nitrogen to produce urea

TRYPTOPHAN IN THE BODY

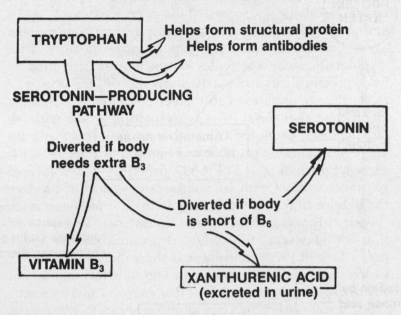

vitamins B_6 and C, together with serotonin. The obvious remedy is to take a free-form supplement of tryptophan together with its vitamin cofactors. Of course, cutting down on smoking and drinking, which contribute to vitamin shortage, will also help.

But tryptophan has another metabolic pathway—a more complex, multistage process resulting in the production of a form of vitamin B_3. This pathway is really a metabolic fail-safe mechanism. B_3 is such an important substance in the body that if normal dietary sources are blocked, the body will use tryptophan molecules to create the B_3 it needs, even if it means diverting tryptophan away from its normal serotonin-producing pathway. So supplying tryptophan, B_6, and C alone might not relieve the insomnia, anxiety, and other symptoms of serotonin deficiency. The symptoms might actually have been caused as an indirect result of B_3 deficiency. Therefore, to cover every eventuality, ensuring that each pathway is as well supplied as possible, you would add a supplement of B_3 to the others.

Now let's follow another amino acid as it reacts in the body's metabolic pathways. This time we'll look at an amino called methionine, a well-recognized antifatigue agent that is also used to help improve memory. Like tryptophan, some molecules of methionine are used to build protein structures, particularly those of the skin. The molecules not used here can then be employed in a number of different pathways. In one, methionine reacts with an enzyme (itself produced from other aminos, together with magnesium) and is transformed into a substance called s-adenosyl-methionine. The body uses this newly formed substance to react with yet another amino acid to produce the fight-or-flight hormone, adrenalin.

After this, the remaining methionine may be converted into one of several substances, depending on the body's needs. One of these substances is the amino acid cysteine, which plays a major role in skin and hair formation, and which may in turn react with other enzymes and cofactors.

So, as you can see, any one amino acid can follow a large number of pathways. Only by following these pathways can we be sure of knowing which supplements to use for relieving a particular disorder. This means taking not only free-form amino acids, but also the vitamin and mineral cofactors that are necessary for ensuring that each conversion stage of the pathway progresses smoothly and efficiently.

3

Getting to Know the Free Aminos

So far we've explored the importance of amino acids as a group of nutrients. Chapter 1 told how they're stripped from the protein molecules in the digestive tract, then distributed as raw materials—building blocks—ready to be reconstructed in whatever form of protein the body needs. Then Chapter 2 described how amino acids, reacting with a variety of enzymes, minerals, and vitamins, create metabolic pathways—the stage-by-stage chemical reactions that run our bodies. And, most important, we've seen how all these pathways can be interrupted by factors ranging from poor digestion, junk food, depression, and stress to viral infection, injury, and poisoning. If one of these factors depletes the body of even a single important nutrient, it can lead to multiple effects as the pathways that need this nutrient are blocked. And, of course, this will in turn deprive the body of other pathway-created nutrients.

If a nutritional deficiency can cause problems, then supplementing the body with missing nutrients can resolve them. But one of the great problems of amino acid deficiency is that it blocks the production of digestive enzymes.

The result of this is to prevent the amino acids contained in the protein you eat from being released. Instead, they sit in the digestive tract and feed bacteria. The resulting putrefaction releases other dangerous substances making the "domino effect" we saw in Chapter 1 radiate outward ever more widely.

Probably the most effective nutritional supplements available today are free-form amino acids. "Free-form" means they are separated from the long protein chains in which they naturally occur. The tremendous advantage of this is that, when you take them, they bypass the need for digestive acids and enzymes and are thus absorbed straight through the intestinal wall. Taking amino acids is like spring-loading each domino—you stop it from ever falling down.

How do you know which aminos to take for particular illnesses and disorders? On the one hand, it's enormously encouraging that health food stores are stocking an ever-growing selection of these extraordinary substances; on the other, most aminos have long, bewildering names, and their containers give almost no indication of how you should use them and for what. For that reason, here is a short introduction to each amino acid.

Strangely, there is no hard-and-fast rule about how many amino acids there are. Some people say 8, others 12, many insist on 20, 22, and even 25. This book will be looking at 18 aminos in particular—those which have been found most effective in relieving a variety of health disorders. Experts generally agree that of these, eight cannot be made by the body, and are thus called the essential amino acids. They are **phenylalanine, tryptophan, methionine, lysine, leucine, isoleucine, valine,** and **threonine.** Recent evidence suggests that **histidine** also cannot be made by the body, so it, too, is an essential amino acid. From the essential aminos, the body can, if necessary, use metabolic pathways to synthesize all the others. Although these amino acids *are* essential to good health, they are called the dietary nonessential amino acids, because if you don't include them in your diet, your body can manufacture them. These amino acids include: **tyrosine**, **taurine**, **cysteine**, **arginine**, **orthinine**, **glutamic acid**, **glutamine**, **proline**, and **glycine**. Be sure you obtain all the nonessential aminos you need, as manufacturing them in the body might divert the eight essential amino acids from meeting other needs.

Don't worry if these names mean nothing to you at the moment. Many of them will appear frequently in the book, and soon you'll be able to recognize their highly individual metabolic "personalities." The following discussion introduces some of the aminos commonly used in dietary supplementation. While this list is by no means complete (and you'll be meeting more as you go through the book), it will give you an idea of how some of the commonly used amino acids work, how they interact with each other.

Note: *Please be sure to read Part Two on the ground rules of amino supplementation before you begin to take aminos.*

ESSENTIAL AMINO ACIDS

Phenylalanine

Phenylalanine is considered an essential dietary amino acid. Normally the body can't make it from other amino components, so you must obtain what you need from your food. Good sources of phenylalanine include beef, chicken, fish, soybeans, eggs, cottage cheese, and milk.

Phenylalanine has several important roles in the body's metabolism. As soon as it is digested and absorbed into the liver, a certain amount is used to build the sugar-regulating hormone, insulin, and other proteins and enzymes. It also contributes to a variety of fibrous protein structures, including collagen and elastin (found in skin and connective tissue).

Note: *Phenylketonurics, or those with PKU, should not take phenylalanine under any circumstances. They and people taking MAO inhibitors or who have high blood pressure should refer to Chapter 5 on "Safety and Precautions."*

Fight-or-Flight Phenylalanine

Phenylalanine acts as the parent molecule of one of the most important metabolic pathways in your body—a pathway that produces a group of hormones known as neurotransmitters. Neurotransmitters are responsible for relaying brain messages from one nerve cell to the next throughout the entire body. The body contains a great many neurotransmitters; some order muscles to contract, others order the body to relax. The particular neurotransmitters created from phenylalanine are called *catecholamines*. When they are released from the nerve cells, they can cause mental arousal and alertness, an elevated and positive mood, and the "fight-or-flight" response to stress. The best known of these phenylalanine-created neurotransmitters is the hormone *adrenalin*.

When the phenylalanine-adrenalin pathway is working smoothly, these substances allow you to cope with stress. Stress is such a continual part of our lives that if this pathway were to become blocked, the stress you'd encounter would quickly overwhelm you, leading to anxiety and depression and later to serious physical illness. So keeping this pathway supplied with phenylalanine and well oiled with its metabolic cofactors is immensely important. Phenylalanine can rouse depression victims, can protect women from the emotionally draining effects of premenstrual tension and menopause, and has even been found to improve learning potential. As it is so important, we'll be examining every stage of the phenylalanine-adrenalin pathway in Chapter 11, "Stresswatch." Because phenylalanine, especially in combination with tyrosine, improves your body's production of adrenalin, it may be inadvisable to take them if you suffer from high blood pressure. The other side of this coin is that people suffering from low blood pressure benefit enormously from using these aminos.

Phenylalanine and the Thyroid Gland

During the first conversion stage of the phenylalanine-adrenalin pathway, an enzyme called phenylalanine-hydroxylase converts phenylalanine to another amino acid, **tyrosine**. (Please note that, since tyrosine can be manufactured by the body, it is a necessary, but dietary nonessential, amino acid as explained above.) A small number of people suffer from a disease that causes a deficiency of the conversion enzyme; the disease is called phenylketonuria (better known as PKU). The deficiency leads to a buildup of unconverted phenylalanine, which means that there is insufficient tyrosine for the production of catecholamine neurotransmitters from L-dopa to adrenalin.

Another result of this enzyme deficiency is that the work rate of the thyroid gland can slow down. The thyroid gland is responsible for the rate of your body's metabolism. It determines how fast you grow and whether the food you eat is stored as fat, burned as energy, or used in the processes of regeneration. It does all this by secreting a regulatory hormone called thyroxin. The amino acid component of this hormone is tyrosine. Phenylketonuria prevents adequate tyrosine from reaching the thyroid gland. The results can be fatigue, obesity, lack of growth, and reduced resistance to disease. All these can be avoided by supplementing the diet with tyrosine, together with the mineral cofactor iodine.

Weight Control

Even those who don't suffer from phenylketonuria can often benefit from metabolic pathways with free-form supplements of tyrosine and phenylalanine with the help of their doctors. This will often stimulate the thyroid gland, increasing the rate of metabolism and thus helping the body to mobilize fat deposits and use food more efficiently. These changes help the patient to lose weight. Another of phenylalanine's actions is to stimulate the intestines to produce a hormone called cholycystokinin (CCK), which tells the brain when you've eaten enough—it helps to curb appetites. So as well as their other benefits, phenylalanine and its partner tyrosine are particularly beneficial when included in a weight-loss program.

Tryptophan

Like phenylalanine, **tryptophan** is an essential amino acid present in most good protein foods (although in much smaller quantities than phenylalanine).

Note: *Persons taking MAO inhibitor drugs should see Chapter 5 on "Safety and Precautions."*

Tryptophan and B Vitamins

Tryptophan was first mentioned as a health aid in 1913, when researchers established a link between the distressing mental illness pellagra and a deficiency of tryptophan. At the time, these results were contradicted by a second group of researchers, who showed that the disease could be treated with equal success by yeast preparations containing no tryptophan at all. It took more than 30 years for experts to realize that the chemical that relieved pellagra was niacin (vitamin B_3).

Niacin can be obtained from sources like yeast, which is why it was found to relieve pellagra. But B_3 can also be manufactured in a metabolic pathway that starts with the amino acid tryptophan. Tryptophan's relationship with B vitamins goes even further. This amino also needs vitamin B_6 before it can be metabolized effectively. You may remember from the previous chapter that a dearth of B_6 causes xanthurenic acid—a form of tryptophan—to be excreted in the urine. Urinary screenings that pick this up not only prove that the body is wasting tryptophan, but also point to low levels of the converting chemical, vitamin B_6.

Tryptophan and Zinc Absorption

Tryptophan is also the parent molecule of a substance called picolinic acid. This is a chemical the body uses to pick up and transport freshly digested zinc molecules through the stomach lining and into the blood. A deficiency of tryptophan, therefore, would also lead to a loss of zinc. Conversely, extra tryptophan increases the body's ability to absorb zinc from the stomach. Zinc is a vital mineral needed to maintain skin and muscle tone, lung elasticity, and enzyme production.

Tryptophan and Anxiety

Perhaps tryptophan's most important role in the body is in the pathway that creates the neurotransmitter serotonin. Unlike the neurotransmitter adrenalin, which works by exciting and arousing the body, serotonin is an inhibitory neurotransmitter, calming the brain and relieving problems such as anxiety and tension. As depression is often the result of an overactive, anxious mind, the soothing effects of serotonin actively work to relieve it. Used in conjunction with the excitory phenylalanine or by itself, tryptophan—as the precursor of serotonin—is a natural and harmless alternative to dangerous antidepressant drugs. Drugs, after all, are substances foreign to your body's chemistry. They force a response. Amino acids, like foods, are natural substances, which allow normal responses to occur.

Tryptophan and Insomnia

Serotonin is also the substance your brain releases to bring about sleep. Tryptophan therefore is a sound alternative to sleeping pills for insomnia. Furthermore, as it works by enhancing a natural metabolic pathway, you won't suffer from any drowsy side effects the following day; during normal waking hours, the body secretes an enzyme that deactivates the sleep-inducing effects.

Tryptophan and Migraines

Tryptophan is also used to relieve migraine. This ability, too, can be attributed to the serotonin-producing pathway, as serotonin has been found to relax muscles and to control the dilation of blood vessels, relieving the pressure areas that cause migraine by distributing the blood more evenly.

Methionine

Methionine is found in most dairy products and meat, but is low in most vegetables and legumes. For this reason, vegetarians will almost certainly benefit from supplementing their normal diets with methionine. Free-form methionine works to improve the tone and pliability of skin, conditions the hair, and strengthens nails that are soft and suffer from easy splitting. **Note:** *Methionine should not be taken without a complementary dosage of magnesium; see Chapter 5 on "Safety and Precautions."*

Sulphur from Methionine

All the aminos we've looked at so far, although important for your physical well-being, are particularly notable, as free-form supplements, for their effects on the brain. They banish depression, increase alertness, assist sleep, and so on. Methionine works by improving the health of your body tissue, because it is a sulphur-based amino acid.

The mineral sulphur is a very important nutrient for our bodies. It protects the cells from airborne pollutants, such as car and airplane exhaust and factory smoke. It slows down the aging process in the cells and encourages the efficient production of protein. We need sulphur for healthy skin, bones, organs, and hair. Sulphur also helps to transport important elements such as selenium and zinc around the body, and, in compound form, has been found to protect the body against radiation. Every day, we use up or excrete about 100 mg of sulphur. Yet even eggs, one of the richest sources of sulphur available, contain just over 50 mg. To compensate, nature has supplied us with a group of four aminos whose molecules all possess sulphur. Besides methionine, they are **cysteine, cystine,** and **taurine** (all dietary nonessentials described later). One gram of free-form cysteine, for example, provides 180 mg of sulphur—over three times the amount contained in an egg.

Methionine and Chelation

Methionine is an excellent chelator, which means that it can locate damaging elements called heavy metals, such as lead, cadmium, and mercury—which are common in the modern urban environment—then literally grab onto them and eliminate them from the body, much like a bouncer throwing an unwelcome drunk into the street. As these metals can lead to hyperactivity, skin complaints, emphysema, other diseases, and premature aging, methionine can be regarded as a most important part of our diets.

Activated Methionine

As we saw in Chapter 2, methionine is also the main component of the chemical s-adenosyl-methionine (essential in the production of adrenalin), for which it also needs adequate amounts of magnesium. S-adenosyl-methionine, also called activated methionine, is widely used in the body's metabolic pathways. When you realize that the phenylalanine pathway needs activated methionine before it can complete its final-stage creation of adrenalin, you begin to see the way that amino acids react with each other in the body. This interdependence—the action of one substance working to strengthen the action of another—is known as synergy. It is one of the reasons for the near-miraculous success of free-form amino acids when they are used in nutritional counseling. Activated methionine has also been found to assist men suffering from the problems of premature ejaculation, and to relieve chronic depression.

Lysine

Lysine is another dietary essential amino acid which, like methionine, is found in negligible amounts in vegetables, grains, seeds, and nuts. Lysine is required to assist in the formation of collagen, the latticework-like tissue that makes up so much of our bodies. It is also present in bone, cartilage, and connective tissue.

Lysine and Calcium

One way in which the body uses lysine is as a carrier molecule for calcium, ensuring that adequate amounts are absorbed through the intestinal wall and distributed to wherever they are needed.

Lysine and Herpes

Tests have shown that lysine suppresses the herpes virus in over 90 percent of those victims who use it. Many are delighted to experience a complete remission. In nearly everyone who uses it, pain disappears overnight, and the resolution of existing vesicles is much more rapid than usual.

Branched-Chain Aminos

The branched-chain amino acids (BCAAs) are a group of three essential aminos—**L-leucine**, **L-isoleucine**, and **L-valine**—that metabolize in the muscles rather than the liver. They are found in nuts and seeds, and a good balance of these three aids wound healing and helps muscle buildup.

Histidine

Histidine sits uncertainly on the borderline between a dietary essential and nonessential. However, since experts cannot identify any metabolic pathway that manufactures it in the body, we put it into the dietary essential group.

Note: *Histidine can sometimes induce early menstruation, and high levels of histamine (for which histidine is the parent molecule) have been linked to schizophrenia; see Chapter 5, "Safety and Precautions."*

Histidine and the Brain

A histidine imbalance results in psychological disorders such as anxiety and schizophrenia, as well as lethargy and fatigue, poor appetite, and nausea (particularly if the victim is pregnant). This is because histidine is the parent molecule of an important and highly active chemical called histamine.

One of histamine's many roles in the body is to act as an inhibitory neurotransmitter. It is used to strengthen the soothing alpha-wave activity of the brain. In this relaxed state, a person is much more resistant to anxiety and stress, able to take problems in stride. If you are histidine-deficient, the lack of histamine unbalances these natural alpha rhythms in the brain, allowing the excitory beta waves—responsible for the brain activity that leads to anger and tension—to dominate. Histidine supplementation helps to prevent this.

Histidine, Immunity, and Allergy

Histidine is also part of your immune response, stored as it is in the highly sensitive group of cells called the mast cells. When the cellular damage caused by viruses, toxins, or allergens affects a mast cell, it bursts to release the histamine to combat the attack. Histamine causes the blood vessels to dilate, leading to the familiar swelling, reddening, and flushing of the skin (which is why anti-inflammatory drugs are called antihistamines). Histamine regulates antibodies, preventing them from overreacting to harmless substances such as pollen and pet fur. This, together with the fact that it is an excellent chelator, makes it one of the best available treatments for autoimmune diseases such as allergies and rheumatoid arthritis.

Histidine and Digestion

Histidine helps to improve digestion by increasing the production of stomach acid. It treats ulcers, and relieves heartburn and the nausea resulting from pregnancy.

Histidine and Sex

Arguably, histidine's most important role today could be in sex therapy. Research shows that the release of histamine from the mast cells is closely related to the physical action of orgasm. Women who are unable to achieve orgasm are usually low in histamine and greatly benefit from histidine supplementation. Alternatively, the problem of premature ejaculation is attributed to excess histamine and, in another example of synergy, can be regulated by using methionine and calcium.

DIETARY NONESSENTIAL AMINO ACIDS

Sulphur-Based Nonessentials

The sulphur-based nonessential aminos are cysteine, cystine, and taurine. If necessary (and if the vitamin and mineral cofactors are present), the body can manufacture these aminos from methionine. However, as this diverts the existing methionine from its own duties—such as converting adrenalin—it's much better to use supplements. Besides their specific benefits, these aminos offer the benefits of their sulphur base. The benefits of sulphur were described under the discussion of methionine.

Taurine

Taurine is one of the most abundant amino acids in the body. It is especially common in the excitable tissues of the central nervous system, where it is thought to have a regulating influence. As such, taurine supplements have been found to control motor tics, including uncontrollable facial twitches, as well as epileptic seizures. Taurine is also used to relieve angina.

Cysteine and Cystine

In the body, **cysteine** will readily convert to **cystine**, and vice versa, so for the sake of convenience we'll refer to either as cysteine. Like methionine, cysteine is a chelator. In cysteine's case it can help eliminate excess copper, which has been linked to behavioral problems. Cysteine is widely used by beauticians as an antiwrinkling agent and it also protects the body from the poisonous effects of alcohol— preventing hangovers, brain and liver damage, and emphysema. It is also used to break down the mucus deposits of illnesses such as bronchitis and cystic fibrosis.

Arginine

Arginine is an immune stimulator and an important component in tissue generation and regeneration. It is most highly concentrated in the skin and connective tissue.

Arginine and Herpes

Since we've mentioned lysine's connection with herpes, we must now bring in the amino acid arginine. While lysine suppresses the herpes virus, arginine has been found to actually encourage it. Therefore when using amino therapy to fight herpes, it's important to keep the ratio of lysine to arginine high in lysine's favor. One way to do this is to take the amino acid ornithine instead of arginine. Ornithine is produced by the first conversion stage of one of arginine's chief metabolic pathways. It is as effective as arginine in stimulating the immune system, yet has no aggravating effect on the herpes virus. See Chapter 5 for more details.

Arginine and Wound Healing

Apart from its relationship with herpes, arginine—or ornithine, if you choose—is one of the most beneficial aminos you can take. While it is considered a dietary nonessential, the body can't manufacture it quickly enough to meet all its needs. Following any sort of wounding, the body always needs additional arginine to repair itself properly. Nutritionists have found that arginine supplements substantially increase the rate of wound healing.

Arginine and Growth Hormone

Arginine is indispensable for optimum growth. It stimulates the pituitary gland into producing growth hormone. This not only speeds wound healing, but ensures that fat is burned more efficiently, while at the same time muscle tissue is being built up. This makes arginine a central part of any weight-reducing program. Many athletes, recognizing how arginine can improve their performances and physiques, include it in their training programs.

Some people have confused arginine with synthetic growth hormones such as anabolic steroids. There is no connection at all. Arginine works simply by encouraging your body to manufacture its own growth hormones which both burn up excess fat and tone existing muscle. Anabolic steroids, on the other hand, can adversely affect many of the body's metabolic pathways.

Arginine and Sperm Count

Many reports suggest that arginine supplements increase sperm count and sperm motility. The high concentration of arginine in seminal fluid confirms this need for arginine, and research shows that an arginine-deficient diet leads to atrophy of the testicles.

Glutamic Acid/Glutamine

Glutamic acid is the most prominent amino in wheat, and it is involved in the metabolism of sugars and fats.

Glutamic Acid and Brain Health

In the brain, glutamic acid combines with the poisonous waste product of metabolic activity, ammonia, to produce **glutamine**. This is a "brain fuel," which affects brain functions—improving alertness, clarity of thought, and mood. In addition to producing this excitory brain chemical, glutamic acid can also produce an inhibitory neurotransmitter called gamma-aminobutyric acid (GABA for short), which has a soothing, calming effect on the brain in much the same way as histidine and tryptophan do. Glutamic acid has already proved valuable in treating mentally retarded patients and victims of epilepsy. Many people use it simply as a pick-me-up.

Glutamic Acid and Blood Sugar

Glutamic acid helps to raise blood sugar and is therefore valuable in the treatment of hypoglycemics (victims of low blood sugar). It has been found to stifle the cravings that many people feel for sweets and alcohol.

Carnitine

Carnitine is actually a dipeptide—an amino acid made from two other aminos. Specifically, carnitine is a product of the essential aminos methionine and lysine.

Carnitine and Fat

Carnitine plays a valuable role in the body, carrying fat into the cells where it is burned to release energy. Once released, this energy increases the body's efficiency, making the physical effort of activities such as sex and weight lifting both more vigorous and more pleasurable. By reducing fat, carnitine helps to prevent heart disease and is an important aid in weight reduction.

Proline

Proline is an important dietary nonessential amino in the protein collagen. (Collagen itself is the most abundant protein in the body.) One-fourth of your body's collagen— which helps make bones and connective tissue—is made of proline.

Glycine

Glycine, like proline, is an important dietary nonessential amino; its molecules make up a third of the collagen in your body. In addition, glycine is important for ridding the body of wastes. If, for example, you drink coffee, the benzoic acids in the coffee damage your cell membranes. They would continue to do this if your body lacked glycine to combine with the acids and form hippuric acid, which is then excreted.

The aminos described here and named in the figure are the most important and regularly used free-form amino acids. Others we'll see occasionally include **asparagine** (aspartic acid), which can be used to alleviate mental and emotional disorders, and **glutathione**, which guards against free-radical (or harmful substance) activity.

MIXING YOUR AMINOS

This chapter has shown how one amino guards against toxicity, another works as a tranquilizer, and a third can improve sexual activity. Yet, as we've hinted, this only gives the barest glimpse of the real health potential of amino acids; the skill comes in using several of them together. For although many people have found relief by taking them

AMINOS AND THE BODY

Lysine. Combats herpes.

Arginine and Ornithine. Can increase sperm count, strengthen immune system, and aid muscle growth.

Histidine. Eases blood pressure. Also helps to relieve frigidity in women and hastens orgasm in men.

Glycine. Reduces sugar craving. Together with *Taurine* helps to relieve diseases such as spasticity.

Cysteine and Methionine. Promote healthy, supple skin and protect from pollution.

Branched-Chain Aminos Leucine, Isoleucine, Valine. Important for muscle growth and repair.

Tyrosine. Important for manufacturing thyroxin, the hormone that regulates the body's growth and rate of metabolism.

Phenylalanine. Precursor of adrenalin.

Tryptophan. Deficiency causes insomnia. Precursor of vitamin B_3.

individually, amino acids work best when they can react in the body with their complementaries. For example, Chapter 12 will provide a formula for relieving anxiety that includes a blend of four aminos—histidine, tryptophan, glycine, and taurine. The different ways in which these aminos affect the body—one calming mental activity, another relaxing you physically, a third easing the overactivity of the excitable tissue—creates a synergy. Unlike drugs or single-strand nutritional support, the effects of this blend as a whole are much greater than the sum of its parts.

Each of the following chapters will address complex medical problems, noting which metabolic pathways are affected, then suggesting what may be the best blend you can take to relieve them. You can effectively use these blends against anything from alcoholism and smoking to allergies, viruses, skin complaints, sexual problems, and more. We'll also list vitamin and mineral cofactors necessary to ensure that the aminos are fully metabolized by the body. If you like, think of cofactors as the metabolic cement for the amino acids' building blocks.

PART TWO
GROUND RULES
OF AMINO
SUPPLEMENTATION

4

How to Use
Amino Acids

If you eat large meals, it can be tempting to imagine that
amino acid supplementation is unnecessary. Western diets,
after all, appear to meet all our body's nutritional demands:
they are rich in fats, carbohydrates, vitamins, minerals, and
especially in proteins—the parent molecules of amino
acids—so why bother with supplementation? The answer is
that although we might actually *consume* all the nutrition
we need, it's unlikely that our bodies will be able to digest
and *use* it effectively. Chapter 1 described how even a simple
toothache can lead to nutritional depletion and illness.

The frightening fact is that our lives are full of such
seemingly innocuous dangers to our health. Smoking,
drinking, stress, pollution, agricultural additives, and eating food that has had much of its goodness processed out of
it can all lead to deficiency-related illnesses, regardless of
how much and how well we seem to eat. Free-form amino
acids, on the other hand, are unaffected by these problems
and will ensure that your body is supplied with all its
essential nutrition. Taken with their important vitamin

and mineral cofactors, they are absorbed easily and provide effective, high-potency nutritional relief.

Once you realize the potential of free-form amino acids in helping to maintain your well-being, as well as relieving existing health problems, the next step is to discover more about them. What are they made from? What quantities should you use? How often should you take them, and when? These are the questions we'll answer in this chapter.

FOOD, NOT MEDICINE

One of the questions most often asked by those wanting to know how much of a particular amino acid they should take is what their "dosage" should be. *Dosage* is a medical-sounding word that gives the impression amino acids are medicines. This is a logical assumption, as people naturally find it hard to accept that something possessing such enormous therapeutic and health-enhancing value isn't a medicine. In fact, free-form amino acids are *foods*—foods in their simplest and purest forms.

People often confuse amino acids with medicines. One woman reluctantly came for nutritional counseling to cure her frigidity. In response to the recommendation of a certain amino acid, she said, "I don't know what I dislike more, this inability to orgasm or having to take drugs to get over it." Like so many others, she simply misunderstood what free-form amino acids are. They're not drugs, and they're generally safe, which is why you can buy them without a prescription in health food stores. They don't work by causing some unnatural change in your metabolism. All they do is help your body to live to its fullest potential.

Note: *There are certain amino acids whose food properties can cause an imbalance in certain individuals, namely phenylketonurics, people with high blood pressure, and those taking MAO inhibitor drugs, in much the same way that sugar can cause imbalance in a diabetic. Refer to Chapter 5, "Safety and Precautions," for details.*

WHAT DOES
"FREE-FORM" MEAN?

The term *free-form* tells you that the molecules of your amino supplement have been extracted—literally "freed"—from the protein chains of foods such as molasses and soy, rather than being created from some complex mixture of laboratory-spawned chemicals. This is good news for all of us who are wary of taking medicines because of the way they suppress the body's natural functions, and is particularly reassuring to vegetarians, as it allows them to use amino acids—the purest sources of protein—without the risk of inadvertently eating meat-based products.

THE BEST FORM OF
AMINOS TO USE

Amino acids come in three forms: the "L" form, the "D" form, and the "DL" form. "L" aminos are utilized in the body directly as proteins; they are easily absorbed and useful biologically. "D" aminos must be converted by the body before they can be used. *Generally, you want the "L" aminos.*

The FDA prohibits the sale of the "D" form, except in two combinations: DL-methionine and DL-phenylalanine (the popular DLPA). *Although I often recommend DLPA for pain relief, I generally recommend against the use of DL-methionine. When taking methionine, take L-methionine.*

Free-form amino acids are commonly sold in the form of 500-mg pills or capsules, although they can also be found in powder form. In powder form, they are usually placed directly on the tongue with a spoon and washed down with a liquid. As the amino acids do not dissolve in water, it is not a good idea to add them to a liquid unless it is something with some body—tomato or apple juice, for instance.

Amino acid supplements are available from retailers under a variety of different brand names. Always ensure that the canister you are buying is clearly labeled with the quantity of "free-form" amino acids, not just "amino acids," it contains. Some manufacturers use cheaply produced protein powder, then include only a small amount of a particular amino acid. A label that indicates a container holds amino acids may mislead a buyer into thinking it is a container of a pure, free-form amino acid.

One of the major advantages of free-form amino acids is that they will be absorbed into the body without having to undergo a lengthy and inefficient process of digestion. If you are misled into taking protein powders instead of amino acids, you will lose this advantage, and you'll end up receiving nutritional benefit only to the extent you are able to digest the protein. Always make sure you know exactly what you're buying; if in doubt, shop elsewhere.

THE IMPORTANCE OF BLENDING YOUR SUPPLEMENTS

As we've seen, each of the fifty thousand or more proteins in your body has its own unique amino acid profile. These profiles are created by metabolic pathways, the stage-by-stage chemical reactions that your body uses to meet its astonishingly long list of needs: transforming aminos into skin tissue, enzymes, hormones, neurotransmitters, hair, and bone structures. Illness occurs when a nutritional depletion blocks a transformation, causing one or more metabolic pathways to work sluggishly. Therefore, when you take free-form amino acids, they help to relieve your illness by unblocking the affected pathways and allowing the transformations to take place.

Different metabolic pathways meet and react with each other all the time. For example, the metabolic pathway that transforms the amino acids phenylalanine into the hormone adrenalin needs to react with an enzyme that has itself been created by a pathway from the amino acid methionine. You should therefore consider not only how taking an amino acid will relieve the blocked metabolic pathway, but also how it will affect the other metabolic pathways that it reacts with.

For instance, imagine that you are under enormous stress at work. To cope, you decide to take a supplement of phenylalanine to encourage your body's adrenalin production. But by doing so, all of your body's methionine is used up in assisting the phenylalanine-adrenalin conversion— methionine that is needed to help other body functions, too. So by increasing your body's phenylalanine levels, you might have unwittingly caused a depletion of methionine. The fatigue that can result from this will leave you just as vulnerable to your work stresses as will low levels of adrenalin.

The key to ensuring that this doesn't happen is to avoid taking one amino supplement on its own. Instead, use a blend of *several aminos together*, such as phenylalanine and methionine when you want to combat stress. This is why, from time to time, instead of suggesting one amino acid to relieve a complaint, this book gives you lists of aminos (sometimes of as many as five or six at once) to take in combination, together with their vitamin and mineral cofactors. These lists are specifically formulated to relieve particular disorders while enhancing the efficiency of any other metabolic pathway that might be affected. Taking nutrients in groups like this is the best possible way of enhancing your body's health and vitality.

DECIDING WHAT TO TAKE

If you've ever noticed that a certain diet, or a certain food, makes you feel better than others, you know firsthand how directly food affects health. Or if you've ever withdrawn a certain food from your diet (say, sugar) and noticed a change in your feeling of well-being, you understand how much food is responsible for overall health. With aminos, the effect is just as great, but you've got to find out which supplements will work for you. You must combine your overall health, your specific symptoms, and the knowledge you have about aminos to come up with the right blends for you.

First check Chapter 5, "Safety and Precautions," to make sure there is nothing in your health profile that would suggest you should avoid certain amino acids. Then read about the basic blend (at the end of this section) and finally read about the aminos recommended for your specific health concerns (Parts Four, Five, and Six). Remember, you'll be taking additional *food*, not medicine; you are, in effect, changing your diet.

If several programs are recommended for your symptoms, pick the one that *best* fits your problem, and begin with that; if you do all of the programs at once, you'll have no idea what's working for you and what's useless! Give it two weeks; if you see no improvement, switch programs, or try adding another to your present regimen. Experiment. You may discover you need several programs concurrently to get the desired results, but work your way up slowly.

Another tip is to try to begin with the program most keyed into the basal *cause* of your problem. With dieting, for example, you'd start with the psychological support program, as psychological dependency is often what causes overeating and overweight.

Evaluate; see what works for you. If you are interested in a more specific idea of what nutrients you lack, there is a urine analysis that can be of great help; see Chapter 6.

HOW MUCH SHOULD YOU TAKE?

It's best to begin with one 500-mg supplement a day of each of the amino acids in your blend—in addition to your complete blend—and slowly increase the amount until you feel them helping you. How much you eventually need to take, and how quickly they affect you, depend very much on your body weight and overall state of well-being. Some people find they have to take as much as 10 grams (10,000 mg) before noticing any benefit, although as a rule, *if you decide to exceed 1,000 mg of an individual amino, it's wise to consult your doctor or a nutritional expert.*

Vitamin and mineral cofactors are sometimes packaged with the aminos; other times you'll buy them separately, usually in pill form.

WHEN TO TAKE YOUR AMINO ACID SUPPLEMENTS

You can take free-form amino acids at any time of the day or night. However, to derive as much nutritional benefit from them as possible, it's best to take them on an empty stomach. This is because if you take them with, or soon after, a meal, they will be forced to compete for absorption through the intestinal wall and in the body with the other, much bulkier, foods. This is a particular problem if you take your supplements with a high-protein meal such as steak or eggs, as these foods will effectively block absorption of your free-form amino acids. Since you want your supplements to be as thoroughly absorbed as possible, it's important to help them to avoid this sort of interference. Therefore, take them at least an hour after any meal and try not to eat for at least half an hour afterward so that your body will have plenty of time to absorb them.

DIGESTIVE SIDE EFFECTS

Since free-form aminos have no fiber or bulk and are absorbed immediately, they may have a mild constipating effect. However, if your diet is rich in fiber—particularly lots of fresh fruit and vegetables—this won't be a problem. Megadoses of amino acids (a very rare 15 grams or more) might cause diarrhea. Finally, aspartic acid may cause flatulence.

HOW LONG SHOULD YOU TAKE THEM?

Some amino acid supplements have been known to show results within 45 minutes. This is especially true of the blends that are designed to enhance your mood and relieve anxiety. Others, taken for their physical effects such as reducing weight and building muscle, take longer. However, no matter what your reasons are for using amino acids, you must be willing to take them for a minimum of two weeks, gradually increasing the amounts during this period, if necessary. You should realize that a deficiency in a certain amino may mean that you will need to take the amino indefinitely, probably in a maintenance, not a therapeutic, level.

5

Safety and Precautions

In their best-selling book, *Life Extension*, Durk Pearson and Sandy Shaw devote an entire chapter to the possible dangers of nutritional supplementation. The chapter, entitled "Is There Anything Perfectly Safe?," consists of one word: No.

The fact is, no matter what you give your body, an element of risk is always involved. Free-form amino acids are the building blocks of protein, and because proteins are part of our daily diets, aminos are very safe. Yet in some patients even aminos may cause the occasional side effect. This chapter recommends a few precautions to follow when taking free-form amino acids and itemizes the adverse reactions that individual aminos have sometimes been known to cause.

TAKE YOUR AMINO ACIDS IN A BLEND

The previous chapter stressed the importance of taking blends of aminos together with vitamin and mineral cofactors, rather than taking them individually. The first, and most important, precaution is simply to try to follow this rule. Taking one amino on its own will not necessarily harm you—indeed, many people benefit immensely from using a single amino acid to help them recover from a disorder. Nonetheless, you should take a blend whose constituent vitamins, minerals, and aminos complement each other, such as those included later in this book.

Perhaps when you imagine the small mountain of supplements you might have to wade through if you follow our suggestions, you'll feel tempted to stick with the small and oh, so convenient bottle of pills prescribed by your doctor. We hope not. Like most worthwhile projects, amino supplementation involves a bit of work and application. After all, the best route toward full health and vitality lies in giving the body an optimal and balanced supply of all it needs, rather than just "pumping up" the area that needs the most obvious attention. This awareness of your body as an interdependent whole, and taking blends accordingly, is the most important and valuable safety measure you can follow.

In general, take the highest quality vitamins and minerals you can find. Talk to your health food or nutritional specialist if you have questions. Do be sure, however, to take "dry," rather than liquid capsule vitamin E, as it does not go rancid.

OTHER WARNINGS AND PRECAUTIONS

None of the following warnings may apply to you, and even if one does, it's the easiest thing in the world to stop taking the offending amino supplement.

Phenylketonuria and Phenylalanine

Note: *You should never take any form of phenylalanine (including DLPA) if you are a phenylketonuric or are on a phenylalanine-restricted diet.* Phenylketonuria is a genetically inherited inability to manufacture the enzyme that converts phenylalanine to tyrosine—the first stage of the metabolic pathway that produces adrenalin. This condition is particularly dangerous during the first four years of life, when, unless the intake of dietary phenylalanine is controlled, this amino will build up and cause mental retardation. However, no matter what your age, *if you suffer from this problem, don't take phenylalanine.*

Other Genetic Disorders

A genetic inability to convert amino acids is a rare problem. However, like phenylketonuria, these disorders do exist, and new ones may be discovered. If you have difficulty metabolizing a particular amino acid, you may suffer by taking free-form amino supplements. You might not even realize you have difficulty converting a particular amino acid until unpleasant physical or psychological symptoms occur. If this happens, stop taking your amino supplements immediately, see your doctor, and start supplementation again only under the direction of your doctor or a qualified nutritionist.

MAO Inhibitors and Phenylalanine, Tyrosine, and Tryptophan

Note: *Avoid the free-form amino acids phenylalanine, tyrosine, and tryptophan if you are taking monoamine oxidase (MAO) inhibitors, the manufactured antidepressants prescribed under many different brand names.* These antidepressants work by inhibiting MAO—an enzyme used by the body to deactivate the stress hormones noradrenalin and adrenalin, and the sleep hormone serotonin, when they are no longer needed. Inhibiting the MAO enzyme allows those hormones to circulate in the body for much longer than usual, so helping to relieve depression, anxiety, and stress. Unfortunately MAO inhibitors can also cause severe depletion of many essential nutrients, and have been known to lead to, among other problems, anorexia.

If you took phenylalanine, tyrosine, or tryptophan (the parent molecules of your stress and sleep hormones) at the same time as MAO inhibitors, there would be a huge surge in the circulating levels of adrenalin, noradrenalin, and serotonin, leading to a range of mood-related and psychotic problems. Because of this potential overload, *you should only take one or the other—either MAO inhibitors or free-form amino acids—never both.* If you are taking MAO inhibitors now, instead of having to forgo amino acids, why not do without the inhibitors? Ask your doctor for advice.

Fears About Tryptophan

Recently, many people have expressed doubts about the safety of the amino acid tryptophan. In addition to the concern over a patient taking tryptophan at the same time as MAO inhibitors (see previous section), concerns have been raised with regard to complications of pregnancy and liver damage.

Pregnancy and Tryptophan

You may notice that tryptophan bottles are labeled with warnings that tryptophan should not be taken by pregnant women. This warning is probably purely a legal safeguard; little evidence suggests that tryptophan is harmful. It is, after all, a dietary essential. We've seen, for example, how the body uses it to manufacture the sleep hormone serotonin, as well as vitamin B_3.

So why the warning to pregnant women? Apparently it stems from a laboratory study published in a medical journal in which a group of hamsters were fed extraordinarily large amounts of supplemental tryptophan as part of their diets. This group produced litters of fractionally lighter birth weight than those of the tryptophan-free control group. Although the tryptophan litters were perfectly healthy in all other respects, companies that manufacture free-form amino acids have been understandably unwilling to repeat these tests on pregnant women while the remotest threat to a safe delivery exists. Instead, they

choose to include a warning to pregnant women on tryptophan bottles as a safeguard. After all, the modest loss of
revenue this might cause is nothing compared to the
damage that could result in a lawsuit from the woman who
happened to be taking tryptophan during her pregnancy
and delivered an abnormal baby.

Liver Trouble and Tryptophan

One other worry about tryptophan is that it has been
rumored to cause liver damage. In particular, it has been
linked to hepatic coma, where the victim's liver loses control
of many metabolic functions, including the regulation of
amino acid metabolism. Some people thought that, because
the levels of tryptophan rise during hepatic coma, tryptophan was one of the causes of the illness. In fact, the excess
tryptophan, far from causing hepatic coma—or any other
liver trouble—is one of the results of the breakdown in
amino acid metabolism.

Despite the current tryptophan scare, there is no direct
evidence to say that tryptophan can harm you. *As always,
however, if you have any doubts whatsoever about taking it,
seek personal advice from an expert.*

Herpes and Arginine

Tests in laboratory conditions suggest that the spread of
herpes can be stimulated by the amino acid arginine. Some
nutritionists feel that in practice it may not stimulate a
spread, as one of arginine's other roles in the body is to
strengthen the immune system against virus infections.
However, *if you have already caught herpes, it's worth
avoiding arginine and substituting ornithine in its place.*
(For details see Chapter 20, "Help Against Herpes.")

Menstruation and Histidine

Consumption of four grams or more of the amino histidine
has been known to cause early menstruation. If you are
using histidine and you find this happening to you, reduce

your intake of the amino, or break the amount you take into much smaller quantities taken more often throughout the day. Some women athletes use histidine to time their periods around important sporting events.

Schizophrenia and Histidine

Histidine is the parent molecule of the highly active substance histamine. Scientists have found a link between high histamine levels and schizophrenia, so *anyone with a history of schizophrenia should seek medical advice before taking free-form supplements of histidine.*

Mental Health and Methionine

Some nutritionists have reported that an excess of methionine may result in psychological problems. This is more probably due to a dietary shortage of magnesium, an important cofactor needed to help convert methionine in the first stage of its metabolic pathway. *Whenever you take methionine, simply make sure that you are also taking supplemental magnesium.*

High Blood Pressure and DL-Phenylalanine, L-Phenylalanine, and Tyrosine

If you suffer from high blood pressure, you should take DL-phenylalanine, L-phenylalanine, and tyrosine—the parent molecules of the fight-or-flight hormones noradrenalin and adrenalin—*only under a doctor's or a nutritionist's guidance. Also have your blood pressure monitored regularly.*

Of the concerns we've addressed in this chapter, it may be that the only safety precaution that applies to you is that you balance your amino intake in a blend, together with vitamins and minerals. In a way, this is less of a precaution than an attitude: when you realize that illness doesn't stem from an isolated case, but an imbalance, you are taking the first step toward a healthier and more vital life.

6

Which Amino Acids Do You Need?

From the start, this book has stressed your body's complexity and sensitivity to change. Variations from an optimal, fully nutritious diet that serves all your body's needs occur very easily. In an attempt to anticipate the disorders that amino deficiencies cause, some enlightened doctors and nutritionists are now using a highly accurate amino acid nutritional test. The test is called a "quantitative urinary amino acid screening." By pinpointing specific deficiencies, this test can often anticipate an illness before it occurs, and in some cases can even show you which aminos you should take to help you avoid it.

It's by no means essential that you have one of these tests conducted before starting to take amino acids. This book is a comprehensive layman's guide to which aminos you should take for which problems. Consequently, you may want to skip over or quickly skim this chapter.

PUT TO THE TEST

A patient who undergoes this test is first required to collect every urination during a 24-hour period. Through the kidneys' natural process of filtering, a certain amount of all the amino acids in the body are spilled into the urine. Analyzing a sample for 40 or more amino acids takes into account the body's full metabolic cycle. From this 24-hour collection, the nutritionist or doctor will find traces of most amino acids. By comparing the amounts contained in these traces with the expected average, the nutritionist can determine whether there are shortages of any aminos, as well as some vitamins, or minerals, and any imbalances or blockages in the metabolic pathways. The test acts much as a metabolic x-ray: identifying the problem, pinpointing the cause, and suggesting a remedy.

The results of this urinary screening are obtained by using a piece of complex technology called a high-pressure liquid chromatography (HPLC) unit. Basically, this device takes each of the aminos contained in the urine and mixes it with a dyeing chemical. The density of the dye color that results depends on the level of the amino in the urine. An electronic eye judges the density and feeds the information into a computer, which then prints out a chart showing the levels of each amino present in the urine.

Imagine your urine sample was found to contain low levels of tryptophan. Knowing how tryptophan affects the body (especially with its serotonin-producing pathway), you could expect to develop symptoms such as depression, anxiety, hypertension, and insomnia, as well as the consequences of zinc deficiency. However, instead of waiting for these problems to surface, you could supplement your diet now with free-form tryptophan, together with the important cofactors of vitamins B_3, B_6, and C and the mineral zinc.

The insights that these tests give into the way that metabolic pathways are blocked and retarded are proving immensely beneficial in helping people to avoid a vast array of nutritionally related problems. They also give the most accurate possible diagnosis of the cause of an illness when it does occur—rather than simply examining the symptoms, which is the common practice. Quantitative urinary amino acid screenings also enable experts to expand their research, as well as to broaden their expertise in the use of amino acids as dietary supplements. More is now known about the individual properties and uses of amino acids than ever before, and this knowledge is rapidly being passed on to the public.

If you decide you would like a urinary screening test, ask your doctor or nutritionist for information about test centers near you. Although amino tests are becoming more and more popular, their availability is still quite limited, and you might discover that there are no facilities in your area. If so, you may want to contact one of the following three laboratories that perform urinary screening tests:

Medabolics (tests and supplements)
573 Hillcrest Drive
Paradise, CA 95969

Smith Klyne Bio-Science Laboratories
7600 Tyrone Ave.
Van Nuys, CA 91405

Doctor's Data
30 W. 101 Roosevelt Rd.
West Chicago, IL 60185

For tests and supplements:
Riner's
1713 Midcrest
Plano, TX 75075
(214) 422-0848

If you would like a screening, contact a laboratory before sending them any samples. Find out their fees for such tests, and also ask for advice on how to ship your urine samples.

SELF-DOSAGE: IS IT SAFE?

Although a urinary screening gives you the most precise indication possible of your nutritional needs, it is by no means essential. With the help of this book, you can develop an effective amino acid program. Many people have expressed doubts about such a free rein: "What if the amino I'm taking isn't the right one for me? Can it be harmful if I don't need to take it?" The simple answer to these fears is to remind you that amino acids are foods. If a free-form amino acid supplement in your blend of aminos and cofactors isn't the one you needed, if your body already has adequate levels of that amino, excess amino molecules will either be broken down by the body and stored or will produce extra energy, with spillover excreted in the urine.

The blends we've recommended in the following pages are listed by symptom. The more you understand about how aminos act and interact to cause these symptoms, the easier it will be for you to determine what you should be taking. Again, if you are at all in doubt, a doctor or nutritional specialist can help you determine which aminos are right for you.

7

Complete Blend, Complete Well-Being

In the course of this book, you'll find that, as well as recommending blends of individual free-form amino acids, we also suggest you include a *complete* amino acid blend in your formula. Many people find that taking all free-form amino acids together in one supplement is every bit as important as taking them individually. Nutritionists agree that it's a valuable nutritional aid in helping to strengthen your resistance to disease (see Chapter 14). More important still is the fact that taking a complete blend of amino acids is a marvelous way of ensuring your overall well-being whether you have been ill or not.

So what is this "complete blend"? The blend is literally a nutritional supplement containing all the commonly used free-form amino acids, ready-mixed in one container. These free-form aminos are blended together in roughly the same proportions as in chicken eggs, (one of the most complete forms of protein found in nature).

You may wonder what the point is of taking free-form aminos individually if you can take a complete blend instead. The answer is that these two forms of amino therapy—complete blend and individual amino—serve very different purposes. When you take a specific formula of two or three aminos, it is to support those metabolic pathways that most directly affect your illness. But in doing so, you should always keep in mind that this illness is likely to have caused a chain reaction of nutritional deficiencies, straining enzyme and hormone production, protein synthesis, and the nervous system throughout the body. Taking the complete blend will help to restore what has been lost through this chain reaction—replenishing and strengthening the body's overall vitality by supplying all its metabolic pathways. Think of the complete blend as a sturdy nutritional foundation on which you can successfully build your more specific, concentrated program to meet your individual needs for amino acids.

Because a complete amino acid blend provides nutritional support for the whole body, many people now take it daily in the same way they would a vitamin or mineral supplement. It works like a nutritional insurance policy, making sure that you have all the digestive enzymes you need, and keeping the metabolic pathways well oiled.

Nutritionists advise a maximum of 10 grams of the complete blend taken three times a day for women, and 15 grams taken three times a day for men, in either pill or powder form. While taking more than 10 or 15 grams a day probably won't hurt you, you won't receive much additional benefit, either. The minimum dosage is usually around 2 grams twice a day, and for best results it should be taken between meals.

When you order the blend from a supplier or buy it in a health store, make sure that this blend is really what the manufacturer claims it to be. Manufacturers can mislead purchasers in several ways. First, they can overload the blend with a high percentage of one of the less expensive aminos, such as glycine. Second, some manufacturers sell what is, more or less, just protein powder with a pinch of free-form aminos added. You want *all* of your supplement to be free-form. And third, manufacturers can sell hydrolyzed protein, broken down chemically or enzymatically, rather than building the blend from free-forms. So watch what you buy! Ideally your complete blend should look something like this:

Aminos:	%
Alanine	2.5
Arginine	9.0
Aspartic acid	2.0
Cysteine	0.5
Citrulline	1.5
Glutamic acid	10.0
Glutamine	10.0
Glycine	3.5
Histidine	2.0
Isoleucine	6.0
Leucine	9.0
Lysine	10.0
Methionine	5.0
Phenylalanine	5.0
Proline	2.0
Serine	5.0
Threonine	4.0
Tryptophan	3.0
Taurine	1.0
Valine	5.0

Taken with the following vitamin and mineral *cofactors*:
    Vitamin B_3
    Vitamin B_6
    Vitamin B_{12}
    Vitamin C
    Magnesium
    Calcium
In addition to helping you stay healthy and at the peak of vitality, the complete blend also makes an essential nutritional supplement for the following conditions:

▶ Acne (see Chapter 22)
▶ Aging (see Chapter 21)
▶ Aid to conception (see Chapter 19)
▶ Alcoholism (see Chapter 25)
▶ Allergies (see Chapter 18)

▶ Anorexia (see Chapter 26)
▶ Arteriosclerosis (see Chapter 16)
▶ Bodybuilding (see Chapter 8)
▶ Brittle nails
▶ Broken bones (see Chapter 23)
▶ Cancer (see Chapter 15)
▶ Cold intolerance
▶ Dieting on a low-protein diet (see Chapter 9)
▶ Digestive problems (see Chapter 17)
▶ Dizziness
▶ Hair loss
▶ Healthy skin (see Chapter 22)
▶ Heart and circulatory trouble (see Chapter 16)
▶ Herpes (see Chapter 20)
▶ Illness (see Chapter 14)
▶ Infection (see Chapter 23)
▶ Injury (see Chapter 23)
▶ Low blood pressure
▶ Pre- and postoperative nutritional support
▶ Shock (see Chapter 23)
▶ Strengthening immune system (see Chapter 14)
▶ Stress (see Chapter 11)
▶ Vegetarianism

PART THREE
AMINOS AND LIFESTYLE

8

Aminos and Bodybuilding

Muscle is a fibrous protein made primarily from amino acids. The demands for muscle protein that intense physical activity places on the body's supplies of amino acids often outweigh the levels of amino acids found in ordinary diets—particularly when they must meet the required increase in muscle bulk caused by bodybuilding. Nutritional supplementation is therefore a vital part of any long-term muscle-increasing program. Without supplementation, the body might be forced to dismantle other existing protein structures in the body in order to provide the amino acids needed for muscle growth, leading in turn to nutritional deficiencies in other, equally important areas of the body. This could result in reduced resistance to infection, emotional disorders, fatigue, and even heart trouble.

THE COMPLETE BLEND

At the moment, the form of nutritional supplementation most widely used by bodybuilders is the common protein powder. However, to provide all the amino acids necessary for muscle growth, the complete free-form amino blend makes much better sense. The complete blend is quickly and easily assimilated by the body, and will circulate directly to areas of the body where amino demands are greatest before being reconstructed as a muscle protein. With the complete blend, a bodybuilder can develop his or her musculature rapidly and thoroughly, safe in the knowledge that intensive exercise is placing no undue and dangerous strain on the body's other protein requirements.

We recommend between 5 and 15 grams of the complete blend both before and after each workout. Bodybuilders who already use this blend find that muscle growth is more rapid and easier to maintain.

GROWTH HORMONE RELEASERS

In addition to the complete blend, more specific combinations of individual amino acids are used for the way they promote muscle growth. Foremost among these are a group of aminos that encourage growth hormone release (GHR). Growth hormone is produced by the pituitary gland and is responsible for maintaining the body at a high level of health. It controls the manufacture of protein, is responsible for long bones and healthy skin and organs, and even helps to burn fat more efficiently. In particular, it strengthens tendons and ligaments and encourages cell uptake of amino acids, and so is vital for ensuring muscle tone. After the age of 30, GHR declines rapidly, and most of the available growth hormone is used simply to repair damage and to aid wound healing.

With the aid of the amino acids ornithine, tyrosine, and tryptophan, the body can be stimulated to produce growth hormone and release it into the body in amounts over and above those needed simply to keep the body healthy. They increase muscle and help to burn excess fat. By increasing the body's production of growth hormone, these free-form aminos can help to build up attractive muscle tissue even when you're sleeping. Two GHR blends are available, one to stimulate the release of growth hormone during the day, the other during the night.

GHR Daytime Blend

Take before and after each workout.
Aminos:
Ornithine
Tyrosine
Cofactors:
Vitamin B_3
Vitamin B_6
Vitamin C

GHR Nighttime Blend

Take just before bed.
Aminos:
Ornithine
Tryptophan
Glycine
Cofactors:
Vitamin B_2
Vitamin B_6
Vitamin C

Some people have mistaken amino acid GHRs for anabolic steroids, the artificial hormones still used widely by athletes. However, there is no similarity at all. Free-form amino acids are foods that naturally stimulate the body's metabolic pathways into working more efficiently; anabolic steroids, on the other hand, have been found to suppress and endanger some parts of the body while artificially heightening its physical performance. They are now banned by many responsible athletic organizations.

MORE MUSCLE BUILDERS

Another important supplement for bodybuilders is a blend

of the branched-chain aminos: leucine, isoleucine, and valine. Most amino acids, once they have been digested, are collected by the liver, ready for distribution throughout the body to meet its innumerable protein requirements. The branched-chain aminos are the exception; rather than going to the liver, they travel directly to the muscles. Because of this, nutritionists have deduced that their main role in the body is to assist muscle growth. Giving the body additional amounts of these three aminos as free-form supplements will help to stimulate muscle growth and immensely increase the benefits of your workout.

Branched-Chain Amino Blend

This blend can be taken together with the GHR daytime blend, before and after the workout—but not with the nighttime blend, as branched-chain aminos hinder the body's absorption of tryptophan.

Aminos:
Leucine
Isoleucine
Valine
Cofactors:
Vitamin B_3
Vitamin B_6
Vitamin C

A BODYBUILDING SUCCESS STORY

The effectiveness of these amino supplements for assisting and increasing muscle growth is demonstrated by Andrew, a regular visitor to his health club. Working behind a desk all day, and a "a bit on the flabby side," Andrew decided to start working out on his club's multigym equipment. "At first I really benefited from lifting weights," Andrew remembered. "After the initial soreness, my muscles seemed to fill out quite quickly, and I felt better and stronger in myself." However, after visiting the gym twice or three times a week for two months, things started to go wrong: "I hit the 'wall.' I'd only have to work out for ten minutes for my arms and legs to feel like jelly; my head would start to ache, and I'd have to stop. At first I thought I was just sick from something, but it continued like this for a couple of weeks. I was ready to give up altogether."

Up to this point, Andrew had not taken any nutritional supplementation, thinking that his three large meals a day were all he needed. In fact, while his diet might at first have met the increased nutritional demands of his workouts, it had become inadequate. Simply eating more meat or eggs to raise his dietary protein levels would have little effect if, because of the overwhelming need for proteins to build his muscles, he had already suffered a drop in the amount of enzymes available to digest his food. If Andrew had continued like this, he would have been forced to take a complete rest from the gym for two or three months every time he felt his strength fade.

Instead, on the advice of a friend who ran a health store at the club, Andrew started following a program of amino-based nutritional supplementation. He decided on a blend of the GHR daytime aminos together with extra amounts of the complete blend. Recently he also started including the branched-chain aminos in his formula. "In no time at all I was back in the multigym and having a ball," he reported. "I found I could work out twice as hard as before, and the muscle growth is constantly improving."

9

The Amino
Dieting Revolution

Carefully selected blends of amino acid supplements make probably the most effective and versatile aids to weight reduction you'll ever find. Most diet programs, while stressing how they will reshape your figure, completely ignore the damage they can cause to the body's hair-trigger-sensitive metabolism. Making sure that the body is adequately nourished while dieting is a concern that rarely enters the dieting equation. The dieting programs offered by amino acids are quite different.

By making your body work more efficiently to metabolize fat and improve muscle tone, their ability to help you lose weight is phenomenal. As the body's essential building blocks, they guard against malnutrition and energy loss. Rather than having to endure the typical dieting grind—the self-denial sustained only by guilt—the increased energy and vigor they release will make dieting an actual pleasure.

Aminos can be used in a variety of ways to help you lose weight. Let's go through them one by one.

FEEDING THE HABIT: THE PSYCHOLOGY OF OVERWEIGHT

One of the most frequent excuses for being overweight is the habit of eating to help you relax or pass the time. At work, for example, you might have a small snack during your coffee break. The physical ritual of unwrapping a bar of chocolate, putting it to your mouth, and chewing it is a convenient way of shifting your mental focus away from work. Many people smoke for the same reason, which is why, if they give up cigarettes, they often substitute food and immediately gain weight.

We also use food as a psychological crutch to cope with anxiety. In our day-to-day lives we experience anxiety frequently—from the demands of a high-pressure job, the anticipation of an examination, or even from fretting over the fate of a soap opera character. Anxiety is a sign that our bodies are reacting to a situation by firing the sympathetic nervous system—the stress response. Eating a snack in these situations is an unconscious attempt to relieve the physical sensations of anxiety. As you chew, and as food passes down into the stomach, digestive enzymes are secreted, blood is pumped away from the heavy muscles, and brainwave activity slows. For evidence, look at cinema statistics. They show that audiences of horror films invariably eat the most popcorn and candy.

The compulsion to eat when you don't really want to—out of habit or in response to anxiety, rather than hunger—is the first problem to tackle when you diet. So start your diet by using the amino anxiety formula:

Aminos:
Tryptophan
Histidine
Glycine
Taurine
Cofactors:
Vitamin B_1
Vitamin B_2

Vitamin B$_6$
Vitamin C
Calcium
Zinc

Taken midmorning and midafternoon (about two hours after breakfast and lunch respectively), the formula helps relieve the anxiety and tension that lead you to eat.

SAY NO MORE: APPETITE REGULATION AND "PLATEAUING"

Many nutritionists and dieters agree that for dieters phenylalanine is the most effective amino of all. This is because it is the parent molecule of three different metabolic pathways, all of which affect your weight. This one amino is practically a weight reduction program on its own.

Let's first look at how it curbs your appetite. Experts have recently found that phenylalanine triggers the release in your stomach of a substance called cholycystokinin (CCK). As far as appetite is concerned, CCK is a hormonal dipstick. When your stomach is empty, CCK levels tend to be very low. This relays a message to the brain, telling you that the body needs food, which you experience as familiar hunger pangs.

Within half an hour of consuming a large meal, the levels of CCK in your stomach have risen by around 50 percent. The new, higher level tells the brain that your body has eaten enough and, as a result, makes you feel physically sated. When you reluctantly refuse that third helping of chocolate mousse at a dinner party, your CCK levels are at their highest. Using phenylalanine supplements to induce CCK release is the perfect way of cutting down the amount of food you eat. Taken last thing at night, many people find that it helps them to avoid those nutritionally worthless, but fattening, midmorning and midafternoon snacks, as well as to choose smaller helpings at mealtimes. Unlike the anxiety blend, which strengthens your mental resolve not to eat, phenylalanine is effective because it makes you feel *physi-cally* full.

The second appetite-curbing pathway involves phenylal-anine's conversion to noradrenalin. This excitory neuro-transmitter, used widely to treat depression, elevates your mood, and reduces your desire to eat.

The third benefit of phenylalanine to your weight reduc-tion program comes from its role as the precursor of the amino acid tyrosine. Tyrosine helps your body to stay at its desired weight once you reach it. This is a godsend for the thousands of dieters who find that staying slim is even harder than losing weight in the first place.

Exactly why is it so difficult, and how can tyrosine help? Well, imagine that by reducing your calorie intake you've lost every ounce you set out to lose. Naturally, you feel delighted. Within weeks, though, the jubilation vanishes as your body inexorably starts to regain the weight it shed.

The responsibility for this disheartening, and very com-mon, reversal lies with the thyroid gland—one of the organs that controls the body's metabolism rate. By secreting the hormone thyroxin, it dictates the extent of generation and growth of every cell in the body, as well as the amount of food burned as energy. To the thyroid gland, your sudden calorie reduction is the equivalent of an army raising a siege. In a siege, the attacking army attempts to starve the defending inhabitants into submission. And in resisting, the inhabitants must conserve as much of their food as they can. Your body is exactly the same. To prolong the existing supplies of food, the thyroid gland secretes less thyroxin, and this reduces the energy-burning metabolism rate. The fact that energy is conserved instead of burned is one reason why you get so tired when you diet.

Several weeks pass. Standing on your bathroom scale, you find you've reached your target. Not wanting to shed any more weight, you relax your eating habits a little. To the embattled thyroid gland, the additional food is wel-come, but the thyroid has no way of knowing whether this food signals an end of the siege or merely a lull between assaults. So rather than secreting more thyroxin to raise the metabolism rate—which will burn the food as energy and increase cell regeneration—the thyroid cunningly maintains the low rate, making the body hoard the food as insurance against further siege. Stored in the body and doing nothing, the food quickly turns to fat, resulting in your dismaying weight increase.

The key to all this is the mischief caused by the low thyroxin levels. Taking it one step further, if you were to raise the amount of thyroxin circulating in the body—thus increasing the metabolism rate—the food you ate would be used to release energy and generate cell repair, rather than accumulating as unwanted fat. This is where tyrosine comes in. For it is this molecule that, combined with iodine in the thyroid gland, produces thyroxin. Supplementing the amount of tyrosine in your body, together with iodine, vitamin B_6, and vitamin C, will provide the materials necessary to raise the natural thyroxin levels.

Taken three times a day—midmorning, midafternoon, and before going to bed—the following aminos will give your body the support it needs to regulate your appetite and metabolize your food instead of letting it sit as unwanted ballast:

Aminos:
Phenylalanine
Tyrosine
Cofactors:
Vitamin B_6
Vitamin C
Iodine

FEEDING THE FURNACES: FROM CHOLESTEROL TO ENERGY

Carnitine is another amino acid attracting attention for the way it breaks down fat deposits in the blood vessels and muscles. Having broken down the fat, carnitine carries it into the cells, where it is burned as fuel. Tests show that the carnitine levels of overweight patients are very low. As a result, they suffer from high blood cholesterol levels, and often from high blood pressure. When the same patients are given a course of supplemental carnitine, their cholesterol levels plummet, and weight loss becomes much easier to achieve.

The energy that is released when the fatty acids are burned also has other benefits. It can lead to increased alertness, greater stamina, and heightened sexual interest. Considering the periods of fatigue that dieters are usually forced to endure, the free energy provided by carnitine is further proof of the advantages of using amino acids.

Carnitine also helps to protect dieters from ketosis. This is the damage caused by an accumulation of ketone bodies—the toxic waste products of fat. When fat is mobilized, ketones are left behind like sediment in a wine bottle. They raise the level of acidity in your blood and make the body dump vital minerals such as potassium, calcium, and magnesium. This can lead to kidney damage and may even be life-threatening if it continues uncontrolled.

To lower cholesterol levels, increase energy, and protect from ketosis: 250–500 mg of L-carnitine daily on an empty stomach.

BATTLE OF THE BINGE: HIGH-PROTEIN DIETS AND THE SWEET TOOTH

A popular method of weight reduction among dieters today is a diet that consists almost exclusively of protein, with as little carbohydrate as possible. There is, however, a serious and largely unrecognized drawback to this type of diet, one that consistently drives would-be dieters to binge on foods with a high carbohydrate content such as cookies and cakes. The cause of the problem lies in a link that connects the levels of tryptophan with the amount of carbohydrate we normally eat.

A tryptophan molecule is large compared with other amino acids. Yet most aminos are distributed throughout the body by the same pathways. This means that the large, cumbersome tryptophan must compete with smaller aminos for absorption through the intestinal wall, and to wherever it is needed in the body. Its sheer size prevents it from being absorbed as thoroughly as the others. One of the immediate effects of a high-protein meal, in which large numbers of amino acids "jostle" for space, is that less tryptophan is able to reach your brain.

Carbohydrates actually *help* you raise your brain's tryptophan levels in relation to other aminos. Keep this in mind if you decide to diet using a high-protein, low-carbohydrate diet; this diet will almost certainly depress your brain tryptophan levels—something that you should always try to avoid.

Why is tryptophan so important? Primarily because it is the precursor of serotonin, and when a high-protein diet depletes tryptophan, the level of this brain chemical drops, too. In previous chapters we've seen that serotonin is a crucially important neurotransmitter. From the brain, its calming, inhibitory action spreads throughout the body, mitigating our response to stress, relieving depression and anxiety, and improving digestion. Most important of all, we need serotonin to be able to sleep and for the way it promotes natural, rhythmic sleeping patterns. By reducing the available serotonin, a high-protein diet works against this. Carbohydrate, on the other hand, simply by encouraging tryptophan pickup, helps to improve these functions.

Not surprisingly then, dieters on a high-protein diet crave carbohydrates. This is a sign that the body is attempting to increase its tryptophan levels. The physical and mental sensations it causes (aggravated by the lack of calming serotonin) can be as tantalizing and as agonizing as withdrawal symptoms. For many people, the impulse to binge becomes overwhelming. The guilt and self-recrimination that follow are meaningless in that first, resigned instant of cloying satisfaction when they bite into their doughnut or Danish pastry. Any resolve simply flies out of the window, together with their diet.

The simple and effective solution to this is to take supplemental tryptophan. Many dieters find that this is all they need to dispel the anxiety and acuteness of their carbohydrate cravings.

Another amino that dieters are finding helpful is glycine. Glycine is the most commonly occurring amino acid in the body. Because of its relatively small structure, it is used as a sort of cement, filling in the spiral structure of collagen, giving this protein structure its resiliency. Urinary amino tests show that glycine levels in victims of obesity are consistently much lower than average. Significantly, glycine has a pleasant, sweet taste, and some nutritionists think that a link exists between the "sweet tooth" of overweight people and a glycine deficiency. Their craving for sweet things is probably caused by the body's efforts to replace the missing glycine.

The help that glycine and tryptophan gave to Don shows how effective they could be in your diet. A divorcé, Don's eating habits were basically good—lots of fresh salads, fish, eggs, and some lean meat, together with plenty of exercise. His problem was that almost every night he would follow his nutritious main course with a huge bowl of freshly baked rice pudding. "It had almost as much sugar in it as rice," he said, "and there was a hell of a lot of rice. It was funny, the more often I cooked it, the more I enjoyed it, savored it. Cooking and eating it was a sort of ritual. If I went out or couldn't be bothered to cook it, I might actually start fretting and fantasizing about it." As he was entering middle age, the excess carbohydrate and cholesterol were making him put on weight dramatically.

When he came for nutritional counseling, it was to find help for his weight, which he felt was starting to interfere with his social life. He was also suffering from insomnia— a sign of how low his tryptophan/serotonin levels were. It wasn't until tests showed depleted levels of glycine as well as the expected tryptophan deficiency that his rice craving came to light. A blend of these two aminos was recommended, together with vitamins B₃, B₆, and C. As he reported later, "I went completely off the thought of those rice and sugar binges. It amazes me now looking at the size of the bowl that I could eat so much of what was obviously doing me so much harm. Hell, it's almost big enough to do the washing up in." His weight dropped considerably, and he's been fine since.

Here's the anti-binge program:

Aminos:

Tryptophan

Glycine

Cofactors:

Vitamin B_3

Vitamin B_6

Vitamin C

BURNING FAT, NOT MUSCLE

Another method of weight reduction centers on the use of amino acids to produce human growth hormones. The terrific advantage of growth hormone release (GHR) is that, in addition to burning off your fat deposits, the hormone actually helps strengthen and tone your muscles. Aminos are responsible for GHR. The most important are ornithine and tyrosine.

GHR inhibits the formation of fat, mobilizing existing fat stores as fatty acids and burning them for energy. Strenuous physical exercise, which saturates the body with oxygen, is one of the natural triggers of GHR, accounting for the superb muscle tone of many athletes. The levels of this hormone are highest in children, which explains why they can eat so voraciously without getting fat.

Growth hormone secretion declines sharply when we are about 30. For most of us, there is just too little GHR to metabolize our fat deposits. This is why amino acid supplements are so important. Orthinine and tyrosine actually increase the levels of growth hormone released from the pituitary. New muscle protein is created at the expense of fat, which is burned as energy. Tensile strength of the structural protein collagen is also increased. This is particularly important to dieters; instead of your skin sagging as you lose weight, healthy collagen will help it to contract to your new shape, retaining its firmness and pliability.

The best time to take the growth hormone releasers is just before going to bed. This is because natural growth hormone secretion usually occurs some 90 minutes after we fall asleep:

Aminos:
Ornithine
Tryptophan

THE FLIP SIDE OF GROWTH

Each day of your life, your body undergoes a complete anabolic/catabolic cycle. The anabolic cycle involves the processes of construction and regeneration, of manufacturing new enzymes and protein structures. It uses up the body's existing energy. The other, catabolic, phase is destructive. It tears down the existing protein structures, dismantles enzymes and hormones.

The aminos the body uses to manufacture growth hormone affect your body anabolically. This is to say the functions they perform are essentially related to growth, to building up and regenerating cell structure.

However, the anabolic/catabolic processes are very complex. Since the body naturally shifts from one phase to the other, you can't treat, or diagnose, an illness based on a single observation. Consider, for example, anorexics and victims of obesity. You would think, naturally enough, that the physical results of an anorexic's obsessive concern with weight reduction—virtually trying to "tear down" her whole body—would be well and truly catabolic. Surprisingly, it isn't. In a near total state of depletion, an anorexic body wedges itself obstinately into a permanent anabolic state, simply as a method of self-preservation. Continuously building itself up with the few resources it has is the only way it can survive. It's rather like trying to stop an incoming tide by using a toy spade to build a sand wall— the only chance you have of preventing the water from sweeping the wall away is to frantically pile more and more sand on top.

While the physical emaciation of anorexia is character-ized by an anabolic response, obesity is brought about by the efforts of a fat body to stave off further weight gain, like a dam opening its sluice gate to prevent the water in its reservoir from overflowing. Most of the amino therapies we've looked into so far are anabolic (phenylalanine, tyro-sine, tryptophan, and the growth hormone aminos). To ensure that the body's own catabolic defenses against weight gain are not disrupted, you can take specific aminos to strengthen your catabolic response:

Aminos:
Methionine
Taurine
Cysteine
Aspartic acid
Glutamic acid
Cofactors:
Vitamine A
Vitamin B_6
Vitamin B_{12}
Folic acid
Vitamin C (as Calcium Ascorbate)
Magnesium Aspartate

Using them to supplement your body at the start of its catabolic cycle—normally at its maximum from 4:00 P.M. until 10:00 P.M.—they will help to tear down the fat you can't see in your blood vessels, muscles, and organs, as well as the fat you *can* see bulging over the elastic of your underwear.

By timing these metabolic phases properly, you are practically introducing a shift system, or relay, of weight-reducing measures into your body. Once the catabolic demolition finishes, the anabolic one will begin, spearheaded by the bedtime supplements of the growth hormone aminos.

The story of one young woman, Marian, who came to us at her wits' end, illustrates the importance of a balanced anabolic/catabolic cycle. She explained that during a year of severe emotional strain—her father's death coinciding with the breakup of her marriage—she had turned to food for support. Quickly she gained an alarming 50 pounds. Finally realizing the danger, she switched to a diet consisting almost exclusively of fresh fruit. Her body rapidly shed 20 pounds; then it stopped. "It just wouldn't lose another ounce," she said. "It's as if it were stuck." What had actually happened was that her metabolic balance, knocked around like a pinball first one way by the weight gain, then the other by the diet, had finally reacted. In an effort to stabilize the fluctuations of weight, it had become permanently anabolic, arresting any further weight loss by continuously building up tissue to compensate. Marian was given a high dosage of the catabolic aminos to take at five o'clock every evening. During the day she took carnitine, and before bed the growth-hormone-releasing aminos, ornithine, lysine, and tyrosine. Her weight began to drop again, and within three months she was back to her original weight.

As Marian discovered, dieting is a battle of wits between you and your body. Even when you do start to lose weight, there is always the danger of being outmaneuvered by the body's hormonal responses. Despite your best efforts, you might inexplicably start to regain the weight you lost or find yourself caught in an irresistible craving for some high-calorie, high-carbohydrate food. Instead of fighting a dreary war of attrition against these things, accept them for what they are—signs that your choice of weight reduction is harming you—and take steps to put things right. This means first and foremost satisfying the nutritional demands

of your body. Using amino acids and their cofactors helps
you to avoid causing dangerous nutritional depletions when
you diet. And by helping your body to work more efficiently—building new muscle, burning excess fat, and
helping to resist cravings—the assistance they give you
might make you wonder how you ever got along without
them.

PUTTING IT ALL TOGETHER

If so many different programs seem a little confusing,
Chapters 4 and 6 can clarify them for you. I'd suggest that
most dieters start with the psychological program, as the
reasons we overeat are more often psychological than physiological. Try appetite control next, then the growth hormone program—see what works best for you.

Part Four
AMINO BRAIN POWER

Nowhere is the potential of amino acids for improving health greater than in the way they assist brain metabolism. The brain is the master control center of your whole body. It consumes 25 percent of all metabolic energy, and the six billion nerve cells it contains make up half the body's total nerve cells. It stimulates motor functions, digestion, growth, and tissue repair; it interprets your sensory experiences and decides which physical and emotional responses to make.

Yet despite this incredible power, your brain constitutes only 2 percent of your body's weight. This makes it highly sensitive: nutritional deficiencies can cause brain imbalances that send shock waves through your entire body, resulting in everything from fatigue and forgetfulness to depression and anxiety. But these disorders can be prevented. By using free-form amino acids together with their cofactors, you can dramatically strengthen the fragile mechanisms of the brain, giving yourself more energy, optimism, and alertness than you ever realized were attainable.

The easiest way to understand the workings of your brain is to think of it as an enormous reference library, containing a mass of highly sensitive and chemically active cells instead of a collection of well-thumbed books. For in the same way that the reference library houses reams of wisdom and learning, so the brain cells are a great storehouse of priceless information for directing the body. It's when something happens to block the distribution of this information that illness, both mental and physical, results.

Every second, your brain receives thousands of requests from its cells to supply information. Such requests arrive in the form of messages brought by the nervous system from every point in the body. The brain's job is to sort through these messages—matching and comparing them with the mass of knowledge it has accumulated through a lifetime of experiences—and find a response appropriate to each of them. If, for example, a message comes from the stomach saying that it contains freshly eaten food, the brain searches through its cells until it discovers how it responded previously to a similar message. Having found a precedent, it sends out a reply ordering the stomach to secrete those acids and enzymes needed to digest the food.

The orders your brain dispatches are incredibly diverse— it tells muscles to contract, your heart to pump faster, your body to go to sleep or snap to excited awareness. These orders are sent from the brain in split seconds from receiving a request for information. In fact, it takes the brain only one-thirtieth of a second to receive, as a nerve message, the bang of a popped paper bag and send out an order to the body to give a start.

We began by calling the brain a reference library. However, a librarian would never be capable of cross-referencing it. The brain contains more than six billion nerve cells (half the total amount for the whole body), and each one shares the information that determines its response with up to ten thousand others. The overwhelmed librarian would have to compile an index containing 60 trillion entries.

This fantastic interconnection is what gives the brain its versatility. With it the brain can run the billions of subconscious reactions that occur daily, as well as provide the conscious functions of memory, inquisitiveness, reason, and emotion. In fact, nothing in your body will work if the brain doesn't. It determines not only emotional and mental states but the energy levels, growth, and general health and functioning of the body. Many of the body's most disturbing illnesses—including Parkinson's disease, Alzheimer's disease, senility, and schizophrenia—are a direct result of brain dysfunction.

Now, thanks to today's metabolic approach to nutrition, neither these nor other brain problems have to be accepted as an inevitable part of our lives. By understanding the relationship between nutrition and brain chemistry, then using amino acids, their vitamin cofactors, and mineral activators to supplement our diets, we can accomplish almost anything. We are biochemical beings whose biochemistry can be influenced nutritionally—for better or worse. And brain changes are not the simple accidents of nature that many people believe.

AMINO ACIDS AND NEUROTRANSMITTERS

The connective mechanism of your brain—the way that one cell passes information to and receives information from the next—is the important element in learning to use amino acid brain therapy. When a message is carried by the nervous system, either into the brain or back to the part of the body waiting for orders, it is transmitted through the nerve cells as an electrical wave. This wave is conducted through one cell at a time, passing to the tip of a branchlike structure on the cell's surface called an axon. From here, the message is transmitted from the axon across the minute space that separates one cell from another—a synapse—to a receiving branch on the neighboring cell, called a dendrite. The message then passes through this second cell to its own axon before crossing to the dendrite of a third cell. The relaying process continues until the message reaches its destination.

What interests us most is the way the message crosses the
space between axon and dendrite: the synapse. It's tempting
to think of this passage as similar to the action of a spark
plug in a car, the electrical wave bridging the gap on its
own. In fact, it doesn't happen like this at all. The wave is
unable to cross this space on its own, and depends on a
special chemical to carry it. This chemical is contained in
a sac at the tip of the axon. The sac bursts as it is contacted
by the electrical wave, releasing the chemical into the
synapse to make contact with the adjacent cell's dendrite.
This contact between chemical and dendrite triggers an
electrical wave in the second cell, which passes through to
the axon on the cell's far side and activates the release of
another messenger chemical—and so on. After its use, the
chemical is either deactivated by enzymes or reabsorbed into
the sac.

Thus, nerve fibers are far from simple conducting cables.
They are in fact a series of relay stations that depend on
special chemicals every bit as much as they do electrical
impulses. A different chemical exists for each type of
message, but collectively these chemicals are called neurotransmitters. Every message to and from the brain needs
these substances. Some affect our emotions, allowing us to
feel happy or angry; others enable us to move, contracting
and relaxing muscles. Often many messages are carried at
once, as in sexual arousal. If we take a mind-altering
drug—be it a sleeping pill, an antidepressant, alcohol, or
LSD—it works by altering the chemical composition of
either the neurotransmitters themselves or their receptor
sites.

Crucially, almost all of these neurotransmitters are made
from amino acids. And there is strong evidence to show that
many of the most important neurotransmitters—such as
adrenalin and serotonin—depend directly on diet. Therefore, by using free-form amino supplements of the amino
acids that make up the neurotransmitters, you can actually
change the nature and intensity of the brain messages they
carry. (The figure gives some examples.) Many mood

AMINOS AND THE BRAIN

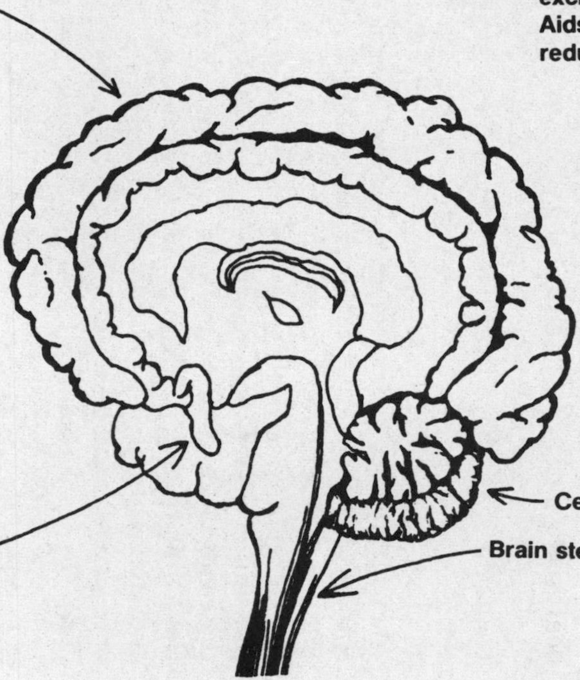

Glutamine. Brain fuel and excitory neurotransmitter. Aids concentration and reduces mental fatigue.

Tryptophan. Precursor of inhibitory neurotransmitter serotonin. Relieves insomnia and combats depression.

Phenylalanine and Tyrosine. Precursors of noradrenalin and adrenalin, which are important for easing depression and stress.

Cerebellum

Brain stem

Cerebral cortex

GABA (Gamma Amino Butyric Acid). An inhibitory neurotransmitter.

Arginine. Helps to improve memory as precursor of spermine.

Histidine. As precursor of histamine, has a powerful calming effect.

Pituitary gland

disorders such as depression and anxiety are inextricably linked with deficiencies or excesses of certain neurotransmitters. For example, without phenylalanine and tyrosine, your brain wouldn't be able to produce all the adrenalin it needs to help you respond to stress. Instead, you would feel torpid, lethargic, and depressed. By providing your body with extra phenylalanine, you can actually relieve the problem.

The following four chapters show how this approach works. Specific blends of amino acids with their vitamin and mineral cofactors give the greatest relief from problems such as forgetfulness, stress, chronic depression, and anxiety neurosis.

10

Alertness and Memory

Some amino acids can be helpful even if you are mentally and emotionally healthy. For example, at times, you may be less alert than you'd like, or you may have days when you find it impossible to concentrate or remember. Amino acids can help with these days.

INCREASING ALERTNESS WITH "BRAIN FUEL"

To maintain efficient brain function, one of the most helpful free-form amino supplements is glutamic acid. Its importance lies in the fact that the body needs it to rid the brain of ammonia—a highly poisonous natural chemical. If allowed to accumulate in the body, ammonia causes irritability, nausea, vomiting, tremors, hallucinations, and eventually death. Ammonia is created in the body by the breakdown of worn-out protein, a natural and continuous process of the body's metabolism. Wherever protein is used—and that means everywhere in the body—ammonia is certain to be present.

The process your body employs to clear this ammonia is

called the urea cycle—a metabolic pathway that converts ammonia to urea, which the body can harmlessly excrete in its urine. The first and most important stage of this pathway is the reaction of glutamic acid with ammonia. The two combine to produce the harmless chemical glutamine. However, if your body has a deficiency of glutamic acid, much of the ammonia will remain unconverted. And the implications of this for the brain are frightening.

As 25 percent of all the body's metabolic activity occurs in the brain, the waste product of this activity, ammonia, will be much more concentrated there than anywhere else. Even a minor shortage of glutamic acid causes the ammonia levels to rise slightly, leading to fatigue, confusion, an inability to concentrate, and exaggerated mood swings— problems that are common to almost all of us at some point. Supplementing with extra glutamic acid helps avoid these symptoms by combining with the ammonia to produce nontoxic glutamine.

There is, however, one problem with taking supplementary glutamic acid. Scientists have found that it doesn't easily cross the blood-brain barrier, a membrane that protects the brain cells from poisons carried in the blood. Glutamine, on the other hand, crosses this barrier with ease. Once in the brain, it will convert to glutamic acid before combining with ammonia and converting back to glutamine. This is why we recommend that you take glutamine rather than glutamic acid.

Once the ammonia has been converted, the brain can use glutamine, like the sugar glucose, as a source of energy. So taking glutamine is almost like plugging your brain into a free fuel source. Not only does it make you feel healthier, it can actually benefit your work. Students, for example, find that taking glutamine supplements in the evening helps them concentrate on homework; they can also work much later into the night without feeling tired. Unlike the caffeine contained in tea and coffee, glutamine stimulates the brain by naturally supporting the brain's metabolic pathways. You feel livelier when you take glutamine because it unblocks the vitality we all possess but rarely release—unlike coffee, which provides an artificial stimulation at the expense of your health. Students have also taken glutamine before examinations. They report greater mental alertness and clarity, and few of the doubts that often surface during exams.

Glutamine is widely used in the United States to combat jet lag. It allows you to travel comfortably for long periods without needing to sleep so that you can adapt much more quickly to local time. Business people are discovering how helpful glutamine can be. One man who came for nutritional counseling, John, works in the foreign exchange offices of a multinational bank in London. He spends most of his day on the phone, buying and selling large amounts of currency. Before transactions, he seeks out information, warily interpreting the "mood" of the international money markets. He must be sensitive to every price fluctuation and trend, with thousands of dollars resting on the outcome of his decisions. It's a highly stressful job.

When he came for couseling, John complained of extreme tiredness at work: "It's as if I knew what I had to do but just couldn't engage my brain," he recalled. "My mind was active in a way that a fly is active when it's stuck to flypaper—all that expenditure of energy and no result. I was getting less and less done and making some pretty bad decisions. Half the time I couldn't care less; the other half I was panic-stricken." John was advised to take glutamine together with cofactors, and the surge in his energy and enthusiasm for work took place overnight: "I felt so refreshed—it was like I was in a state of constantly having just stepped out of an invigorating shower."

If you feel lethargic and confused, find it difficult to concentrate, lack enthusiasm, or just feel in need of a pick-me-up, try this blend three times a day:

Amino:
Glutamine
Cofactors:
Folic acid
Vitamin B_6
Vitamin C

MEMORIES ARE MADE OF THESE

Another common and annoying problem is loss of memory. How often have you seen a face and been unable to put a name to it, or vainly tried to conjure up a specific word or the title of a film? Have you ever left on a trip only to freeze in panic when you couldn't remember whether you'd turned off the oven or closed a window? For most of us, this forgetfulness is only a minor frustration. For some it is deadly serious. The chronic forms of memory loss are presenile (occurring before 60 years of age) and senile (occurring after 60) dementia. In their acute stages they leave victims with little awareness of who they are or of their surroundings, unresponsive to those around them and often incontinent. Now, as a result of research into the severest forms of this distressing illness, amino acids are being used not only to help these, but even the milder forms of memory loss that we all experience.

This research—much of it conducted in the seventies by Carl Pfeiffer at the Brain Bio Center in Princeton—found that the one factor all senility patients had in common was low levels of a substance called spermine in the blood and brain. Spermine is a product of the amino acid arginine and is found in semen, blood tissue, and brain cells. When Pfeiffer examined people with good memories, he found their spermine levels to be many times higher than those of the senility victims. It seems fairly certain that when the levels of spermine in your body drop, your memory becomes impaired.

The theory put forward to explain how spermine deficiency impairs memory is quite complicated. It goes back to the production of ribonucleic acid (RNA). The body uses RNA to duplicate sections of the master blueprint—DNA— whenever tissue needs to grow or to be repaired. The DNA selects the number and assortment of substances that are needed to make a particular section of tissue. In addition, it seems that RNA in the brain cells is also important for storing our memories.

RNA is made by an enzyme called RNA polymerase, and this enzyme is activated by spermine. Insufficient spermine will lead to a deficiency of brain RNA, in turn causing a loss of memory. Therefore, raising spermine levels increases the production of RNA and actually helps to improve your memory.

Spermine is produced from arginine by a complicated metabolic pathway involving several cofactors. All these nutrients must be included in any memory-enhancing formula, so let's look at the pathway to see how it works. It starts when arginine reacts with an enzyme activated by manganese to produce the amino acid ornithine. Reacting in turn with vitamin B_6, ornithine is converted to putrescine. At this point, activated methionine—itself created from magnesium and methionine—converts putrescine first to spermidine and then to spermine. If you want to help the pathway progress smoothly—and to improve your memory—try a blend of nutrients taken once or twice a day between meals:

Aminos:
Methionine
Arginine
Ornithine
Cofactors:
Vitamin B_6
Vitamin C
Manganese
Magnesium

Note: *Arginine should not be taken by herpes sufferers; see Chapter 5, "Safety and Precautions," for more information.*

11
Stresswatch

By now most people realize that uncontrolled stress brings trouble, contributing to insomnia, gastric ulcers, high blood pressure, asthma, migraine, and many other problems. Prolonged or excessive stress is also considered a major factor in premature aging and the development of degenerative diseases. Stress will strip your body of essential nutrients like a thief in a jeweler's shop. Unfortunately, with the high-pressure demands of our society, continual contact with the factors that cause stress—called stressors— is inevitable. What we *can* do is to use amino acid supplementation to dramatically strengthen the body's ability to cope with stress when it occurs.

But what *is* stress? A climber clinging uncertainly to the face of a cliff feels stress. So do children waiting for a school bus in the freezing rain and a homemaker who burns a hand on the stove. Their specific reactions vary: The climber sweats and gets a tight stomach, the children go pale and shiver, and the homemaker suffers an inflamed hand and emotional shock. However, their internal biochemical responses are the same. They all undergo the increased production of the neurotransmitter adrenalin, and this leads to other biochemical, neurological, and physical changes that help them cope with the increased demands on their bodies. These reactions are called the stress response. It always takes place in exactly the same way, regardless of what has caused the stress.

Severe physical exhaustion, surgery, and starvation diets can cause great stress. However, stress isn't brought on only by extreme physical conditions. Emotions we all experience—anger, fear, frustration, excitement—are stressors. So are allergic reactions to food or the environment, infections, degenerative and chronic debilitative conditions, and even insomnia. All of these stressors are so much a part of our daily lives that we take them for granted.

Understanding the stress response and the biochemical changes it effects is important. It will show you how to improve your ability to cope with stress by providing your body with the nutritional support it needs. This in turn can improve health, balance emotions, and prevent premature aging and degeneration.

THE STRESS RESPONSE

While people's specific responses to stress are as varied as the number of stressors they encounter, the biological nature of this response is similar in every case. It is called the *general adaptation syndrome* (GAS), and its purpose is to preserve life by maintaining stability in the body's structure and function, a condition called *homeostasis*. Every stressor disrupts homeostasis to some extent. When this happens, GAS comes into play. It has three stages: alarm, resistance, and exhaustion.

The *alarm stage* is responsible for our "fight or flight" instincts. To meet the increased biological demands, the brain waves change, blood flow increases to the muscles, and adrenalin is released more quickly. These changes are known as the sympathetic nervous system response.

In the *resistance stage*, the body's systems are mobilized to meet the threat of the stressor. This stage can last for a long time or a short time, depending on the intensity of the threat. The longer it continues, the more vital nutrients will be depleted in sustaining the resistance.

The body rarely gets to the *exhaustion stage* of GAS. But when it does, the weakest systems break down, and chronic fatigue and illness follow. The exhaustion stage seldom continues, except in cases of extreme shock or old age. However, if it does, the result is eventually death.

To see the kind of biochemical demands that stress makes on your body, consider the metabolic reactions necessary to sustain the alarm and resistance stages of GAS. This is what happens:

▶ Protein breaks down, especially in the muscles.
▶ Fat is mobilized.
▶ Salt is retained, and minerals such as potassium are lost.
▶ Synthesis of liver protein slows, kidney function is impaired, and immune functions decline, leading to fatigue and susceptibility to illness.
▶ Amino acids are stripped from the body and consumed as a source of energy to meet the heightened metabolic requirements of stress. These amino acids are needed elsewhere in the body.

This is the kind of violence that prolonged stress does to the body's natural biochemical balance. And although your reaction to stress in normal circumstances may be only a fraction of this, your metabolic balance is slowly but surely being chipped away by the effects of ordinary, everyday stress.

Each of us differs in how much stress we can take before reaching the exhaustion stage. This depends partly on conditioning—to what extent we can become at ease with something that at first is stressful—but also on our level of nutritional support. With optimal levels of supplementation, we can withstand a lot of stress; faced with the same stress, but with inadequate nutrition, we quickly reach exhaustion.

You can use amino acids and their cofactors to strengthen your basic vitality and resistance to stress, so that you stave off the exhaustion stage of GAS. You need more than one or two nutrients; you need a whole family of aminos, vitamins, and other cofactors that enable your body to respond well to stress. To understand why, look at how each nutrient is involved.

THE BIOCHEMICAL RELAY RACE

A primary function of GAS is release of adrenalin—the driving force of the stress reaction. It is the fuel that powers your body's rise to the demands being made on it. This important hormone is produced by a metabolic pathway beginning with the parent amino acid phenylalanine. Considering the many nutrients needed to complete this process, it is worth describing the reaction step by step to show how important each nutrient is, and how dependent they are on each other.

The whole process of stress response resembles a relay race. A relay team's victory depends on the speed of each runner, the smoothness of each baton pass, the state of the track, and each runner's fitness. In the case of the stress response, the finishing line is the production of adrenalin. The starting gun is fired when the parent amino acid, phenylalanine, reacts with an enzyme called phenylalanine-4-monooxygenase. This produces the amino acid tyrosine. Tyrosine is acted upon in turn by the enzyme tyrosine-hydrooxylase and becomes L-dopa, another amino acid. At this stage, vitamin B_6 and phosphorus, acting together as cofactors, convert the L-dopa into the catecholamine neurotransmitter dopamine. The complex nature of the whole process is reinforced when you realize that this reaction also requires the presence of adequate magnesium. The next stage is the production of noradrenalin from dopamine. This can occur only when dopamine reacts with vitamin C and copper. Finally, to convert noradrenalin into adrenalin, your body needs the activated form of methionine, s-adenosyl-methionine.

What all this means is that when you are taking nutrients as a biological support mechanism—either for general health or a specific healing process—it is vitally important to focus on the entire family of nutrients, rather than expecting results from just one or two. If even a single nutrient is in low supply on the stress pathway, the biochemical relay will become sluggish, and the body will suffer by receiving inadequate amounts of adrenalin.

REDUCING STRESS

The message of all this is simple. When the metabolic relay from phenylalanine is not flowing as it should, then your body's response to stress is inadequate. This is a widespread phenomenon in the West, as are its symptoms of fatigue, lowered resistance to illness, depression, and premature aging. The process can, in effect, remove all the sparkle from your life. That's the bad news.

The good news is that by supplementing your body with the free amino acids, vitamins, and minerals needed for the stress response, you often can easily and surprisingly alter your whole experience of life and health. And despite the great complexity of interrelated metabolic pathways involved, this task is not overwhelmingly difficult. In essence, it involves examining these metabolic pathways, noting the particular substances involved, and supplying them through your diet together with wisely selected nutritional supplementation.

Let's briefly look at the nutrients involved in the specific stress-related metabolic pathways. The figure illustrates where these nutrients come into play. From this information, we can outline the foundations of a metabolic nutritional program that is the basis of high-level health and effective holistic amino acid supplementation.

Let's start with protein breakdown. The destruction of protein during stress produces increased quantities of ammonia. The body can only get rid of this poison through the urea cycle by consigning this waste into the urine, which is then eliminated from the body. The function of this particular metabolic pathway is maintained through the amino acid glutamine.

METABOLIC PATHWAY
OF THE STRESS RESPONSE

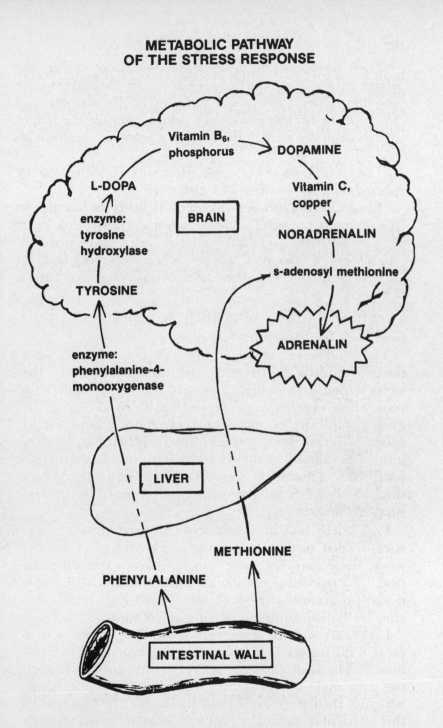

Then, to support the heavy demands made on the thyroid gland during stress, the body needs the amino acid tyrosine and the mineral iodine. Combining in the thyroid, they produce the hormone thyroxin, which controls the rate of metabolism not only in the body as a whole but in individual cells.

The actual production of adrenalin is facilitated by phenylalanine, tyrosine, and methionine.

The following combination of nutrients is the foundation for the most powerful antidote to stress known to science. Use it whenever you find yourself under heavy demands from work or emotional worries, when recovering from an illness, or at any other time when stress becomes a burden for you.

Take three times a day between meals:

Aminos:
Glutamine
Phenylalanine
Tyrosine
Methionine

Cofactors:
Vitamin A
Vitamin B_1
Vitamin B_2
Vitamin B_6
Vitamin B_{12}
Vitamin C
Vitamin E
Pantothenic acid
Choline
Folic acid
Niacin
Magnesium
Potassium
Manganese

Note: *Before taking these nutrients, see Chapter 5, "Safety and Precautions."*

12
Anxiety—Not All in Your Mind

Stated simply, anxiety is a stress response. Its symptoms—quickened heartbeat; the taut, queasy sensation in the stomach; perspiration; and heightened mental alertness—are all part of an alarm system. Your body is warning you of a stressful situation, and these uncomfortable sensations are caused by its efforts to respond. This anxiety response is vital. It prepares us for activities that need increased physical or mental effort and even warns us away from others. It is usually short-lived. One person in twenty, though, suffers from a continual, unreasoning dread that psychiatrists call anxiety neurosis. It can inflict severe physical degeneration on victims and leave them mentally unable to face the demands of life.

What causes this extreme response? The best way to find out is by looking at a classic cause of anxiety. Then, once we understand the psychological and mental problems involved, we can formulate an amino acid blend to fight it.

ANXIETY: CAUSES

Imagine sitting in your car at the red traffic light of an

intersection. The light changes to green. You've repeated these actions so often that you release the brake almost unconsciously, ease your foot off the clutch, and press the accelerator. The car moves forward. Suddenly another car, running a red light, slams into your side. You are treated for shock and a few cuts and bruises, but all things considered, you feel lucky to be alive.

A few weeks later you come up to the same intersection. Again the light is red and the memories of the accident come vividly to life: the screech of brakes, the thundering concussion as the cars hit, tossing you sideways, the breaking glass. Now, instead of the easy, reflexive way you usually move off, you are acutely conscious of your actions. You realize that it was exactly this chain of events that led to the accident and that every movement you now make is repeating the chain. The light changes and your throat tightens, your palm is sweaty on the gearshift, and your movements are tense and jerky. The car moves off, and you grit your teeth, your senses alert to danger.

The chance of being hit a second time in the same circumstances is almost nonexistent. But the point is that the accident has conditioned your mind to fire the stress response whenever a similar situation arises. This sort of unrealistic fear is the source of anxiety. Our lives are full of the conditions that cause it. Perhaps as a child you were punished for sleeping in class, so that whenever you relax now you always feel guilty about it. Or you might have once been bitten by a dog, leaving you terrified of all dogs. Anxiety might even be caused by a quite unrealistic fear, such as the threat of failing a job interview.

ANXIETY: EFFECTS

However irrational the causes, your anxiety results from fear: of being late for work, of public speaking, or of crashing your car. When we are frightened, our bodies elicit the stress response, releasing adrenalin. Heartbeat increases; nostrils dilate; blood is diverted to the heavy muscles; and the high-frequency beta waves in the brain increase, shifting it to a state of greater alertness, watching for danger. And the low-frequency alpha waves associated with mental tranquility diminish; the mouth becomes dry; secretion of digestive enzymes slows down; and blood is moved away from the intestines. This rapid change accounts for the familiar sensations of anxiety: the roller-coaster feeling in your stomach, the slight trembling and clumsiness of your muscles as they prepare for action, and the acute alertness (like the person afraid of flying, who notices each subtle change of pitch in the noise of the jet engine).

Most of us occasionally experience minor symptoms of anxiety—even if it's only from watching a football team we support play an important game. For some, though, even this anxiety is intolerable. Their sense of dread at the outcome makes it impossible for them to watch. On a wider scale, the normal, everyday challenges of their lives become harder to face, forcing them to draw back from their responsibilities and shirk confrontation.

Alleviating anxiety means having to rebalance the stress response naturally, using specific amino acids to strengthen the inhibitory nervous system. Or you can use Valium—and live as best you can with the side effects as it unbalances other metabolic pathways. If you decide on the aminos, there are four in particular that relieve anxiety so successfully they are often prescribed as a blend. We'll look at each in turn and see how they work.

THE AMINO ANXIETY FORMULA

Histidine

The first of the four is histidine—the parent molecule of the highly active amino acid histamine. One of histamine's many functions is to act as a neuroinhibitor, reducing the intensity of beta waves in the brain and encouraging the growth of alpha-wave levels. When histamine levels are low, your alpha-wave levels subside. The result is the sort of irritability, uncertainty, and mental confusion we associate with anxiety. But by taking histidine supplements, you can promote the alpha-wave functions, calming and relaxing your mind when anxiety threatens to take a grip.

Histamine also helps to increase the production of gastric juices in the stomach. This offsets the digestive problems that anxiety causes, including severe indigestion and stomach ulcers.

Sarah's case shows the importance of histidine. She is a 36-year-old computer programmer who sought help because of her anxiety. She was generally fit and followed a good nutritional program, but she found that the high-pressure demands of her job were starting to make her irritable and confused toward her work and her friends. Formerly proud and confident of her professionalism, she started to give way to self-doubt and an acute fear of failure. "My ease with my work had flown out of the window," she said, "and I thought everyone around me was conspiring to get me sacked for my incompetence. When my manager asked me questions, I was so scared about fluffing the answer that my throat constricted and all that came out were little gasps."

A urinary analysis showed that, compared to the other amino acids in her body, her histidine levels were extremely low. A daily dose of supplemental histidine was prescribed, and after taking it for only two weeks she reported a tremendous improvement. Her old confidence and assurance had returned, and she was able to look back on her period of anxiety with amused disbelief.

Tryptophan

The second amino in our blend is tryptophan. As the precursor to the inhibitory sleep-inducing neurotransmitter serotonin, it helps to relieve anxiety simply by helping you to relax. When anxiety patients are tested, their serotonin levels are usually found to be depleted. This depletion plays a large part in making you overreact to the stimuli in life (like perspiring and gritting your teeth as you watch that ominous traffic light change from red to green). Depletion also influences the barely concealed aggression you may feel toward a person who, quite innocently, causes you to feel anxiety. And if your brain has too little serotonin, you simply won't be able to sleep. Extra tryptophan can help to overcome all these difficulties. And, unlike the dosage for depression, which has to be strictly limited, you can take it during the day.

Tryptophan is also the precursor of vitamin B_3. All B vitamins are crucial for mental and emotional balance, and serious deficiencies can lead to depression, schizophrenia, and paranoia. A lack of B_3 in particular may cause the nervousness, irritability, and apprehension we associate with anxiety. As the psychologist Abram Hoffer observed, "If all the B_3 were removed from our food, everyone would be psychotic within a year." In their book *Psychodietetics*, Drs. Cheraskin and Rindsdorf tested the balancing effects of tryptophan on 66 volunteers. Those taking the highest doses of tryptophan (over 100 mg) described a remarkable increase in their mental composure and an almost total disappearance of anxiety.

Glycine

The third member of the alpha-wave-producing blend is glycine. Glycine acts as an inhibitory neurotransmitter, but unlike histamine and tryptophan, which react in the brain, glycine works by inhibiting the nerve cells in the spinal cord. In other words, we need it to help control our motor functions—the way our bodies move. Research is showing that glycine deficiency results in jerky, exaggerated movement and sometimes even spasticity. Recently researcher P. Stern gave glycine to seven spastic volunteers. Of these, six were delighted to find that the glycine dramatically eased their spasms and contractions, as well as improving their overall muscle tone.

How does this help your anxiety? Well, think back to your feelings as you sat in your imaginary car when the light changed to green. You know that last time, in these identical circumstances, the car crashed. The light changes, and you fumble for the brake, pressing down so timidly on the accelerator that the car almost stalls. All these movements you usually take for granted are suddenly uncoordinated and magnified. It's as if your body isn't yours at all but a new one that you're learning to use. Now forget the car and think of the last time you personally felt extreme anxiety. You probably reacted in the same way. Although short-lived, this loss of control is similar to the effects of spasticity, which we know can be treated with glycine. Glycine works by inhibiting the messages from the spinal cord that cause these abnormal responses. Taking glycine supplements can eliminate the defective muscle control that, during anxiety, makes every movement a nightmare of self-consciousness.

Taurine

A similar rationale exists for including the fourth amino acid of the blend, taurine. Taurine is a simple sulphur-containing compound and one of the most abundant amino acids in the body. It is found in especially high concentrations in the excitable tissues such as the heart and skeletal muscle. The central nervous system also carries large amounts. Much of the research conducted into the uses of taurine centers on its function in nerve tissue and its inhibitory action on epilepsy. After an epileptic seizure, the nerve tissue where the attack was centered shows very low levels of taurine. Considering the generally high concentrations elsewhere and the fact that epilepsy, like spasticity, is caused by a dysfunction of the inhibitory neurotransmitters, researchers assumed that the attacks generally occurred where levels of taurine were low. Since then it has been found highly effective in reducing seizures, and it is included in the formula for its powerful inhibitory action.

A well-formulated blend of free-form amino acids and cofactors should contain the following:
Aminos:
Tryptophan
Histidine

Glycine
Taurine
Cofactors:
Vitamin B$_1$
Vitamin B$_2$
Vitamin B$_6$
Calcium as ascorbate
Vitamin C
Zinc

You will need to experiment to find exactly how much suits your metabolism, taking between two and ten doses of this blend a day. **Note:** *Before taking any aminos, review Chapter 5, "Safety and Precautions."*

All in all, anxiety is an unnecessary, almost superstitious fear. When you move off from that fateful intersection, you know rationally that you won't be hit again. But how do you convince your racing heartbeat, your sweaty brow, and your suddenly uncoordinated limbs? Simple: Whether you use them to help you stop grinding your teeth, or to relax you before an important interview, this blend of amino acids makes the gentlest, but firmest, of metabolic persuaders. Use it wisely, and you may never balk at a red light again.

13

Depression—A Brain Symptom

Depression is a paradox. Think of it: The most spectacularly able thing known to humanity—your brain—brought low by an overwhelming sense of futility and uselessness, a belief that life is just too difficult. The Healing Research Trust describes classic full-blown depression as "the loss of capacity to enjoy life, combined with a poverty of thought and movement."

Depression is the common cold of mental disorders. One person in a hundred suffers from it right now. And if it has never affected you, there is a better than one-in-eight chance that it will.

It's easy enough to glimpse the numbing effects of depression. Picture yourself on a family outing. It's a Labor Day weekend, and you've driven into the country. But the sky is lead gray, and sleet spatters horizontally across the windshield, reducing everyone to a sense of despondency and lethargy. Conversation is held in bad-tempered monosyllables, and even drawing a face on the fogged window requires a huge effort. You want to drive home, but it just doesn't seem to matter enough to bother.

We've all found ourselves in situations like this, feeling

nothing but despondency and blind to the mass of future possibilities. Of course, once the sun comes out, we'll remember the Frisbee in the trunk, and the world will be fine. Some people, though, continually live in this state. This condition is called pathological depression. It strips the sufferers of their sense of self-worth and leaves them feeling inadequate and unresponsive. Often their mental disorder leads to physical illness—sometimes suicide.

Let's examine the specific causes and effects of depression. Then, by seeing which metabolic pathways are involved, we can formulate an amino-based nutritional program that frees the mind from depression's deadening grasp.

CAUSES AND EFFECTS OF DEPRESSION

Depression can occur from an unexpected stressful event in life—the death of someone you love, for example. The sudden and prolonged stress this causes quickly depletes your body of vital nutrients, resulting in fatigue and torpor, to the extent that it might hardly seem worth making the effort of rousing yourself.

A 67-year-old man we know, whose wife died recently, slept for six weeks in his living room. This wasn't for fear of the memories that sleeping in his bedroom would bring— the shock of his bereavement simply left him without the energy or mental focus to contemplate climbing the stairs. The same thing may happen if you lose your job, fail an important exam, or separate from your spouse or lover.

When depression lacks an obvious cause, doctors have difficulty treating it and it often becomes chronic. It might be characterized by intense self-hate, apathy, spontaneous crying spells, lack of mental focus, and a craving for solitude. A depressed person may even be bewildered by the ability of others to show enthusiasm for activities and ideas. And because of the sufferer's indifference to recovery, this condition is often self-perpetuating.

The depressed person's indifference toward personal well-being also makes him or her neglect proper diet. The result is nutritional deficiency. The more the body is starved of vital nutrients, the less able it is to cope with the demands placed on it. Before long, the body spirals downward on a widening course of illness and degeneration.

Depression is difficult to prevent because its effects may often be delayed, or hidden in other symptoms. And it's difficult to treat because a depressed person often doesn't care whether or not he or she recovers. However, if we can uncover the biochemical imbalances that cause depression, we can use amino acids and their cofactors to correct these imbalances. Let's start with the most important cells in the body: the nerves.

THE NEED FOR NEUROTRANSMITTERS

To relay the brain's electrical messages from one nerve cell to the next, the nerve endings (axons) must secrete neurotransmitters. Certain neurotransmitters carry pain sensations, while others order voluntary muscle movement; some cause excitory emotional responses, others are inhibitory.

The neurotransmitters that govern our excitory emotional responses are called catecholamines—noradrenalin and adrenalin, derived from the amino acids phenylalanine and tyrosine. Our reactions to everything we encounter—the way we are stirred by a piece of music, angered by an argument, amused by a joke—depend on the body levels of these specific neurotransmitters. Too much or too little of any of these substances will make us under- or overreact, according to the stimulus.

Many psychologists and nutritionists are convinced that depression is caused by deficiencies of the catecholamines, with poor nutrition and digestion as the culprits. This spotlights the enormous advantage of free-form amino acids. They don't need to be digested, but are circulated straight to the areas of depletion to provide immediate relief.

But if nutrition is important for treating depression, why

do victims so often end up on the psychiatrist's couch? The last thing a psychiatrist considers is the patient's possible malnutrition. The answer is that, until quite recently, many people thought that the production of neurotransmitters in the brain occurred independent of diet. This was because of protective cells in the brain called the *blood-brain barrier*.

The Blood-Brain Border Patrol

One of the many roles of the blood is to collect water-soluble toxic wastes from the cells and carry them to the liver and kidneys for excretion. On its journey, the blood is pumped through the brain, delivering oxygen and removing carbon dioxide. However, if the toxins that it carries with it were allowed to come into contact with brain cells, the effects would be catastrophic.

Instead, as the blood is channeled into the minute branched capillaries of the brain, oxygen is filtered through a sheath of special cells on the capillary wall. These cells form the blood-brain barrier. Like a border patrol, they identify and reject the toxins that attempt to enter with the oxygen. The toxins continue to circulate in the blood until they reach the kidneys and liver, which send them out of the body.

Because the brain is the last organ to suffer depletion when the body starves, the blood-brain barrier was also thought to protect the brain from harmful changes in diet. In other words, we could eat as little or as much as we liked without affecting brain functions. We now know this is not true: our eating directly affects our production of neurotransmitters. And, because neurotransmitters determine our mental and emotional well-being, it follows that we can help correct depression nutritionally.

AMINOS AND DEPRESSION RELIEF

Several amino acids are involved in making mood-influencing neurotransmitters. Let's now see how they can be used to provide deep and lasting relief from depression.

DL-Phenylalanine

Perhaps the most important and effective amino acid for treating depression is DL-phenylalanine (DLPA). It works better than the more commonly used L-phenylalanine, because it is able to prevent the breakdown of endorphin hormones, the morphine-like substances produced by the adrenal gland (along with the catecholamines) in times of stress. Endorphins are the body's natural painkillers; they cause the euphoria experienced by athletes as they pass through the "pain barrier." They also provide immediate and dramatic relief to depression victims.

To be effective, endorphins must be injected either into the spinal column or the brain itself, a dangerous treatment. Moreover, enzymes break them down quickly, so that any relief is short-lived. DL-phenylalanine blocks the action of these endorphin-destroying enzymes, allowing the antidepressant effects of the endorphins to last much longer. And, rather than the body adapting to DLPA and needing progressively more DLPA to block the endorphin-destroying enzymes, the beneficial effects actually accumulate and become stronger with time.

DLPA also strengthens the nerve-cell metabolic pathways which produce the excitory neurotransmitters noradrenalin and adrenalin. If your body produces enough of these hormones to meet its needs, it can better withstand the stresses that cause depression (such as bereavement). But if your cells are depleted—by poor digestion, perhaps—they won't be able to charge up the brain when stresses occur.

One of the first chemical causes of depression to be identified was catecholamine deficiency. Many of today's antidepressant drugs work by preventing the reuptake of catecholamines in the nervous system. Unlike the natural stimulating effects of DL-phenylalanine, however, synthetic antidepressants can lead to serious and harmful side effects: Though these drugs elevate noradrenalin and adrenalin release to elevate your mood, they prevent them from being reabsorbed by the nerve terminals. The next time catecholamines are needed, the cells are placed under increased stress to yield more without the support of protein reinforcement. The store of noradrenalin and adrenalin can become exhausted, resulting in nausea, seizures, and anorexia.

The advantage of DLPA is that even as it stimulates catecholamine release, it strengthens the whole metabolic pathway. The nerve cells are allowed to perform naturally. They reabsorb their neurotransmitters after use, which prevents the harmful deterioration caused by synthetic drugs.

Tyrosine

The production of noradrenalin and adrenalin is only part of the stress response. The fatigue and apathy of depression often occur when the body is unable to respond to stress demands. Levels of the fight-or-flight hormone, adrenalin, are nearly always negligible in depression patients. The entire pathway therefore requires nutritional support. Along with DLPA, you should take the amino acid tyrosine. Tyrosine is a product of phenylalanine and, as it is one step along the metabolic pathway that leads to adrenalin, it encourages the stress response.

Methionine

The final stage of the pathway—converting noradrenalin to adrenalin—requires s-adenosyl-methionine to affect the change. And the amino acid methionine is the precursor of this molecule. It also removes excess histamine. This is important because histamine is an inhibitory neurotransmitter and can easily contribute to a patient's depression if it is present in the body in excess. Many persons who still suffer chronic depression despite good nutrition are delighted to find that adding methionine to their diets solves this problem.

If you are suffering from depression, try taking this combination of nutrients up to three times a day:

Aminos:
DL-phenylalanine

Tyrosine
Methionine
Cofactors:
Magnesium
Vitamin B_1
Zinc
Vitamin B_3
Vitamin B_6
Vitamin C

Note: *A word of caution: Do not take tyrosine or any form of phenylalanine if you are also taking MAO inhibitors. See Chapter 5, "Safety and Precautions," for more information.*

The following case illustrates the importance of using nutritional supplementation to support the stress hormones noradrenalin and adrenalin. During a period of ten years, a patient we'll call Rachel had become progressively more tired and depressed. Finding it hard to exert herself, she eventually decided to give up her job at a firm of management consultants. At home, her relationship with her husband seemed equally fruitless, but she simply felt too apathetic to try to change anything. In the face of her almost total unresponsiveness, and seeing no prospect of improvement, her husband left her. "It was a terrible time," she said. "I could always see what needed to be done, but there was this massive blanket of inertia holding me back." Things got worse as she was forced to take a part-time job to support herself and her young son. Conserving all the energy she had for the job, she withdrew completely from any social contact. Finally, she decided to come for nutritional counseling. A urinary amino acid test showed that the phenylalanine and tyrosine levels in her body were almost nonexistent. She was given supplements of these aminos and their cofactors and showed an immediate improvement. She felt more positive, suddenly found herself full of energy, and soon started making plans to renew her life.

As these supplements all work on the same metabolic pathway, they create a synergistic overlap; the effects of one treatment complement the effects of the others. This accounts for their effectiveness in treating depression. Recent double-blind tests (where neither the researchers nor the subjects know who is receiving what) have shown that DLPA is at least as effective as the most commonly prescribed antidepressant—and without any of the harmful side effects. It is also widely used to relieve mood disorders associated with premenstrual syndrome.

PERCHANCE TO SLEEP

Once depression has a grip on you, the mental and physical fatigue that results is one of its most unpleasant symptoms. But despite near-total exhaustion, you will find it is impossible to sleep. And lying awake in the small hours, your thoughts fragmented, is a desperate experience. This acute insomnia is caused by a deficiency of the inhibitory neurotransmitter serotonin, the chemical responsible for making us sleep.

Serotonin's precursor is the active amino acid tryptophan. But the body also needs tryptophan elsewhere to create vitamin B_3. As the nutritional deficiencies of stress and depression compound themselves throughout the body, large amounts of tryptophan are withdrawn from the serotonin pathway. The result is a draining, insurmountable exhaustion. Some hospitals treat this problem by knocking their patients out with drugs, feeding them whenever they wake up, then sending them straight back to sleep. Patients are kept in this state for three days.

If you don't like the idea of lying flat on your back in a hospital for 72 hours, your body pumped full of synthetic tranquilizers, try tryptophan. Tryptophan supplements restore your ability to sleep by strengthening the serotonin-producing pathway. People taking tryptophan 20 minutes before retiring find the time taken for them to get to sleep is easily cut in half. And psychologists have discovered that tryptophan has the same antidepressant effects as drugging a patient for days on end, without the harmful drug-induced side effects.

You must be careful not to take too much, though. Serotonin is an inhibitory neurotransmitter that is also used to treat anxiety, a highly alert mental state and virtually the opposite of depression.

Take this formula 10 or 20 minutes before going to bed:
Amino:
Tryptophan
Cofactors:
Vitamin B_3
Vitamin B_6
Vitamin C

Note: *Do not take tryptophan if you are also taking MAO inhibitor drugs. See Chapter 5, "Safety and Precautions."*

RELIEVING SHORT-TERM DEPRESSION

Two aminos that are particularly good for perking you up if you find yourself suffering from short-term depression are glutamine and proline. A man who had become so depressed he had actually tried to kill himself was given glutamine. "I can't believe it," he said after taking it for less than a week. "Is this all I have to do? I feel great. It's changed my life."

Proline gives many people a sense of relief and happiness; others it actually makes angry. Either way, it can elicit a positive emotional response, giving depression victims the momentum they need to recover.

Try this formula three times a day:
Aminos:
Glutamine
Proline
Cofactor:
Vitamin C

Depression narrows our view of life, convincing us that everything is futile, that no effort is worth making. Often, simply by giving in to these feelings they become a self-fulfilling prophecy. But they needn't be. They are, after all, only a small part of our personality, unnaturally inflated by nutritional deficiencies. We all have the potential to be active and productive, and more than any other form of therapy, amino acids can help us tap that potential.

PART FIVE
PATHWAYS TO VITALITY

14

Master Protectors Against Illness

Chapter 1 compared the functions and structures that make up our bodies to a city—a city teeming with a diversity of races and occupations. The inhabitants of your body-city devote themselves selflessly to its upkeep and maintenance. They are fiercely selective about who they allow in and what they use for building materials. To this end, all-seeing, ever-present forces scrutinize every new arrival and keep a watchful eye on the current inhabitants. They are constantly alert to anything that might slip out of place or pose a threat to the overall well-being of the whole. And when a danger is perceived, the defending forces stamp it out, more efficiently and thoroughly than any totalitarian police state.

These brutal-sounding metabolic vigilantes are, in fact, the various constituents of your immune system. They guard against the constant barrage of would-be invaders (viruses, fungi, bacteria) and work to slow down the aging process hastened by factors such as ultraviolet light and pollution-generated free radicals. When one of these factors manages to breach the defenses of your immune system, it starts to break down the complex protein structures of your body's cells and disrupts the metabolic pathways. You experience this breach of your immune system as diarrhea, allergies, colds, vulnerability to debilitating viruses such as herpes and hepatitis, colitis, ulceration, cancer, premature aging, and other disorders. Future chapters will scrutinize many of these problems and show how blends of amino acids, by strengthening individual metabolic pathways, can be used to fight them.

IMMUNITY AND THE COMPLETE BLEND

Every cell, every hormone, and every organ of your immune system is made from protein. So taking the complete blend—even when you're not ill—will provide it with nutritional support to strengthen its function and efficiency. Although individual aminos are used with astonishing success to relieve specific disorders, this complete blend is truly the master protector against illness.

Having the Stomach for Fighting

The first line of your immune defense system against the literally millions of illness-causing organisms that besiege your body is the gastrointestinal system: your stomach and intestines. Here, your body secretes the acids and enzymes that not only digest your food but protect against fermentation, putrefaction, and the buildup of harmful toxins. As with the rest of the body, the gastrointestinal system is a fragile mechanism, balancing between incredible efficiency and chronic illness. For example, to help it digest food, the large intestine—the colon—actually contains vast numbers of potentially harmful bacteria and strains of yeast. It is only the body's own enzymes that maintain the body's control over these organisms: given the chance, they would multiply uncontrollably, causing disease and illness. Unfortunately, with increasing consumption of processed food, this is exactly what is happening.

Fresh fruit and vegetables contain enzymes that help to

limit the growth of the bacteria in the intestines. But processing the food destroys many of these enzymes, straining the body's own enzymes. And so the bacteria and yeast population in the colon explodes, with harmful consequences. With so much yeast, the food actually starts to ferment. The resulting alcohol is absorbed into the blood, the body reacts by lowering its blood sugar levels, and the victim begins to feel tired and rundown. At the same time, the membranous wall of the intestine starts to lose its integrity—undigested protein seeps through into the bloodstream. The body will only accept constituent amino acids, so it reacts to the presence of foreign protein with a painful allergic response—like a small-scale version of the body rejecting an organ transplant or skin graft.

There's more. The oxygen in the intestines, which is needed for digestion, is consumed by the multiplying bacteria, and the putrefaction that this causes produces dangerous toxins which escape into the bloodstream. They roam the body, replacing active neurotransmitters with inert chemicals and blocking metabolic pathways. One particularly virulent form of yeast is called candida albicans. Nutritionists in the United States are worried by the growing number of cases of people suffering from concentrated levels of this yeast in their colons. Evidence suggests that it can cause everything from arthritis to high blood pressure.

What must you do to make sure this never happens to you? Well, since disastrous yeast growth can result from enzyme depletion, the best way to ensure yourself against this is to raise the levels of enzymes in the intestines. Eating unprocessed food will help to a certain extent. But if your digestion is already impaired it will need more than good food to help it recover. Try taking the complete amino blend. At least fifteen thousand enzymes in the body are each the product of metabolic pathways that occur in the pancreas from various amino acid precursors. By providing these precursors to the pancreas in the complete blend, you can help raise the levels of intestinal enzymes, and so reduce the amount of undigested food available to bacteria.

Free-Radical Protection

The amino-derived enzymes also help to guard your body against free-radical damage. Free radicals are unstable molecules, found in polluted air and water. Unlike most molecules, in which the atoms bond by pairing up their electrons, free radicals carry an unpaired electron. In their search for an extra electron, these molecules gluttonously consume the electrons of other, balanced molecules such as those in healthy tissue. This tears apart the protein structures of skin and organs, and causes formerly healthy molecules, in turn, to go in search of electrons to replace the ones they lost, thereby causing illness and degeneration. Heavy metals and ultraviolet light cause a great deal of the free-radical destruction wrought in the body. Amino acids are particularly suited to protecting the body from free radicals, as they latch on to free radicals such as heavy metals and pair them without affecting healthy tissue.

T-Cell Defenses

Another benefit of the complete blend to your immune system is that, as constituents of protein, amino acids are involved at every level in the function of the *endocrine system*. This is the group of glands that includes such glands as the thyroid, the gonads (sex organs), the pituitary, and the adrenal gland.

The different glands secrete different hormones. The adrenal gland secretes adrenalin, which alters the rate of the body's metabolism and prepares the body for fight or flight. The thyroid secretes a hormone called *thyroxin*, which is responsible for food metabolism and repair. Other hormones include the pregnancy hormones FSH and LH, and the pituitary-secreted growth hormone. However, the gland that plays the major role in your immune response is the thymus gland. By linking a number of amino acids and cofactors, the thymus gland produces a hormone called *thymosin*. When this hormone is secreted, it orders the spleen, together with the lymph nodes (small glands situated around your body), to manufacture T-cells. These cells defend against harmful substances.

Imagine the T-cell response as an army, divided into regiments of cavalry, infantry, and heavy artillery. Looking at each "regiment" at a time, the cavalry are those T-cells called lymphocytes. As the army's vanguard, they circulate rapidly around the body, reconnoitering the territory, always looking out for foreign invaders. They are extremely mobile, taking advantage of the interrelationship of every part of the body with every other part. A T-cell can easily travel from a brain cell to a cell in your little toe in its search for infection. It uses the main arteries and veins of the circulatory system before slipping into smaller blood vessels and finally down into the capillaries. From there it will cross to the cell wall. Once it makes contact with the wall, the T-cell will examine it for signs of damage or infection. If the coast is clear, it will leave the cell to travel elsewhere.

When lymphocytes locate an invader, they call up other regiments of their T-cell army. The first to arrive is the infantry, a group of amino-derived hormones called lymphokines. These are thought to be the body's own natural drugs, and include the well-known chemical interferon. They battle microorganisms and toxic chemicals, breaking them down into harmless parts the body can dispose of. If the invader is larger, then the heavy artillery is brought into action: the macrophages. Literally translated, *macrophage* means "big eater," and this is exactly what it does, engulfing the invader and then secreting an enzyme to destroy it.

To work effectively, the T-cells depend on a healthy circulatory system. Not only are blood vessels their main means of transport, but the blood also supplies the thymus, spleen, and lymph nodes with the nutrients they need to function. Victims of heart disorders and obesity, and heavy smokers and drinkers, often find themselves the prey of minor but irritating infections. In each case their circulation is blocked either by a buildup of fat deposits, hemorrhaging, or loss of pliability in their blood vessels. Alcohol also hardens the cells, blocking the T-cell's passage. And as even moderate drinking and smoking impede the immune system, few of us are as healthy as we could be.

This is why the complete blend is so useful. Amino acids are the main constituents of collagen, the flexible protein structure that ensures the pliability of every blood vessel and capillary. Supplementing the body's natural resources of collagen with the complete amino blend helps to maintain its resiliency. This helps lymphocytes reach the area of infection more rapidly. Furthermore, every T-cell—lymphocyte, lymphokine, and macrophage—is made from amino acids (with the help of vitamins, particularly vitamin C and the B complex vitamins).

Antibody Defenses

The T-cell response is one branch of the body's internal defenses. The other is known as the B-cell antibody, or immunoglobin, response. B-cells are made in the bone marrow from amino acid chains, and tryptophan is particularly important for this. There are five groups of antibodies, each of which reacts to a different threat: one to bacteria, another to viruses, a third to toxins, and so on.

They work by joining with the invading substance to render it harmless. An active and mobile germ, for example, might find itself coated with a second skin—the antibody—which insulates it from any contact with the body's cells. Often when the antibody has rendered the invading substance ineffective, a T-cell such as a macrophage will complete the process by breaking down the combined substance.

In fact, T-cells and B-cells often function together in close cooperation. In addition to the three T-cell regiments, there are also two "high commands"—one known as *helper cells*, the other called *suppressors*. When T-cells encounter an invading substance, they produce additional helpers, and these act as a signal, stimulating the production of B-cell antibodies. Suppressors, on the other hand, keep the rate of antibody production to a minimum when they are not needed. The ratio of helpers to suppressors is regulated by substances called *prostaglandins*, which metabolize in a metabolic pathway from a substance called *linoleic acid*, a chemical constituent of fatty acids. As with every metabolic pathway, this linoleic-acid-to-prostaglandin pathway needs amino acids to help prevent blockage.

THE YIN AND YANG OF METABOLISM

The next important function of the complete amino blend is that it supports the natural metabolic rhythms of your body. Every aspect of life is governed by opposing forces—action and reaction, yin and yang, work and rest—and your body is no exception. As Chapter 9 explained, your body passes daily through an anabolic/catabolic cycle of building up and tearing down.

While at first the anabolic phase might seem healthy and the catabolic dangerous, they are both indispensable to our vitality and well-being. Although it's true that we must be able to grow and regenerate existing tissue, it's also necessary to be able to tear down old, worn-out tissue so that the body can build anew. A builder who wants to put up a new house first must totally clear away the vestiges of the old. The body is no different. In a healthy body, these two phases are balanced and help guard against illness. For instance, the growth of skin or hair is a desired, anabolic process—but the growth of a mole is also anabolic, and not very desirable. Cancer, too, is an anabolic process—but the body is usually protected from it by the tearing-down action of its catabolic phase.

An American expert in this field, Dr. Emanuel Revici, conducted detailed research into this area in the early sixties, concluding that many of the illnesses we experience result from an imbalance of this anabolic/catabolic cycle. For example, he found that viruses tend to grow when the body is in a predominantly anabolic state. Bacteria, on the other hand, flourish in a putrefactive—breaking-down—environment, and do best in a catabolic body. Most illnesses, in fact, thrive in one cycle or the other. Revici carried his work further and found that certain food molecules are themselves anabolic, while others are catabolic. Researchers have since conducted a detailed examination of a variety of nutrients to see how they affect these cycles. In the case of amino acids, while most affect the body anabolically (helping tissue buildup), one group is catabolic, assisting the body in its tearing-down process.

The implications of this for your health are immense. As we shall see in following chapters, using amino acids to tilt the body's anabolic/catabolic balance can help you to relieve heart problems, fight viruses, and do much else besides. Taking the complete amino blend will help to maintain the metabolic balance of your body, resisting viruses and bacteria alike and in turn removing stresses from your immune system.

15

Cancer and
Amino Acids

Of all the diseases that afflict humankind, cancer is traditionally the most widely feared. The mere mention of the
word is enough to provoke a shudder, implying an unavoidable and painful death. However, the truth is very different.
Major advances are being made in the field of cancer
prevention and cure through diet and it's certain that free-
form amino acid supplementation will play an ever-growing role in this area. Let's see how amino acids are being
used today to fight cancer.

CANCER AND
THE COMPLETE BLEND

It's often said that cancer victims do not die from the cancer
tumor itself, but from the protein starvation that the cancer
causes in the rest of the body. Amino acids that are used to
build vital protein structures in a normal, healthy body are
instead consumed by the ravenous cancer cells. This bodywide loss of amino acids profoundly affects ordinary body
functions, almost all of which depend for their well-being
on amino acids. Muscle growth and replacement and

wound healing slow down or stop altogether; enzyme and hormone production decline—in turn affecting digestion, the smooth progression of metabolic pathways, and even mental and emotional balance.

Perhaps the most important body function to suffer amino acid loss, though, is the immune system. All the immune fighters of the body—T-cells, antibodies, white blood cells, and so on—are primarily composed of chains of amino acids, amino acids that are devoured instead by the cancer tumor.

So what good can free-form amino acids possibly do? First, they can help to make up for the catastrophic protein loss caused by the tumor. Simply putting the patient on a high-protein diet is not a solution: the stomach would have little chance to digest the protein, due to a shortage of amino-derived digestive enzymes. And what nutrition the body was able to release from the protein meal would simply be gobbled up by the cancer. This is a Catch-22 situation: the body needs protein to survive, but whatever protein you give it acts to strengthen the disease that is killing it.

One answer to this nutritional paradox, many nutritionists agree, is to provide the body with extra large doses of the complete free-form amino acid blend (see Chapter 7). The amino acids will be thoroughly absorbed into the body through the gastrointestinal tract, regardless of the body's digestive shortcomings. While some might be absorbed into the cancer tumor, there will certainly be enough left to strengthen the immune system. The amino acids will also help regenerate enzyme production, which not only means that digestion will improve, but that the body will actually be able to start attacking and tearing apart the cancer tumor. Growth and wound healing will also be resumed on a meaningful scale.

Experts recommend using the complete amino acid blend to supplement a diet high in raw foods. The natural enzymes in raw foods assist the body's digestion. Cooked foods, on the other hand, and meats in particular, lose most of their enzymes in the heating process. This places a much greater demand on the body for digestive enzymes, forcing it to divert aminos that could be used more productively elsewhere in the body—such as helping to strengthen the immune system.

INDIVIDUAL AMINOS

Certain individual aminos are also used in the cancer fight. These include arginine and the constituents of glutathione.

Arginine and the Thymus

Because the thymus gland directs the immune system, it plays a key role in determining the effectiveness of the immune response to cancer. When the body is under attack from cancer, protein loss causes the thymus gland to shrink, thus reducing the strength of the body's immune response. Supplements of free-form arginine, acting as the precursor of growth hormone, increase the size and health of the thymus. This in turn raises the level of thymosin secretion, and the immune response becomes more vigorous. In tests on mice, scientists have found that arginine supplementation inhibits the growth of cancer tumors and often reduces their size.

Extra Defenses Against Cancer

The amino glutathione is also a valuable supplement for fighting cancer. It works as a free-radical scavenger, removing poisons and pollutants that can cause or aggravate cancer. Since glutathione is composed of three separate aminos, it tends to be attacked by digestive enzymes in the stomach; nutritionists therefore believe that supplements of its three constituent aminos—cysteine, glutamic acid, and glycine—would be effective in fighting cancer.

THE CANCER PREVENTION FORMULA

A good, basic cancer prevention program would consist of the following formula:

Aminos:
Complete blend
Arginine
Cysteine (be sure to take cofactors B_6 and C)
Glutamic Acid
Glycine
Cofactors:
Vitamin A
Vitamin B complex
Vitamin C
Vitamin D
Magnesium
Calcium
Selenium

These supplements must be taken in fairly high doses to combat cancer's ability to consume protein. *For this reason, it's important to consult with a doctor or nutritionist before embarking on your program.* **Note:** *Be sure to review the safety precautions in Chapter 5.*

16

The Amino Answer to Heart Disease

A heart attack is a metabolic thunderbolt. Until the instant it strikes, its victim usually feels in excellent health. He or she might not drink, or even smoke. He or she might be as strong as a horse and exercise strenuously. (Of course, this person may admit to occasionally growing very hot and unaccountably short of breath, while insisting it is nothing really to worry about.) Driving to work one morning, and reaching for the gear shift, his or her arm suddenly feels as if the blood in it has turned to lead. Before there is time to wonder what's wrong, a jolt of pain shoots through the arm from shoulder to wrist, and an incredible, relentless, vicelike grip crushes his or her chest, making breathing impossible. Out of the blue, his or her heart stops beating. Even with today's medical expertise, more than 50 percent of deaths in Britain and America are heart related.

The health and efficiency of your heart and circulatory system—more crucially than anything except your brain—depends on a balanced lifestyle. Unfortunately, because of the way we systematically abuse our bodies, few of us enjoy this optimal lifestyle. Smoking and drinking alcohol are obvious abuses. They rob the cells of oxygen and vitamins, raise the levels of toxicity in the body, damage our organs, and lead to high blood pressure.

But your heart can be hurt just as seriously by other, far subtler, problems. Even if you don't smoke or drink, even though you exercise regularly and follow a low-cholesterol diet, you could still suffer a heart attack. A history of poor digestion or nutrition, emotional problems, stress, even inherited disabilities, all make you vulnerable. If they lead to a deficiency in your body of only a small number of vital nutrients, this might be all it takes. Over the years (and heart attacks don't usually occur until the victim is well into middle age), the effects of these deficiencies will accumulate like the effect of a pebble falling down a hill, which eventually causes a landslide. If a molecule needed to create an enzyme is missing, the metabolic pathway that uses this enzyme will be converted much more slowly than it should be. This, in turn, will starve the body of other specific nutrients. In the end, the deficiencies will become widespread and highly damaging—nowhere more so than in your heart.

Heart attacks are usually attributed directly to cholesterol buildup. Even when this is the obvious case, the fact that the victim's body is unable to break the cholesterol down efficiently points to widespread enzyme, vitamin, and mineral deficiencies and not just to a fatty diet.

So treating heart problems isn't only a question of cutting out certain foods. You must actually increase your intake of the nutrients that supply your body's relevant metabolic pathways. When doctors search for the cause of heart problems, though, they ignore these unique biochemical processes. Instead, they look to high technology to enforce a "cure": sophisticated bypass surgery costing tens of thousands of dollars; "piggyback" heart operations and pacemakers; lasers to burn out the debris from blocked arteries; and, most incredible of all, the mechanical replacement hearts connected from the chest by wires to an outside power source. Then, to make the body accept these things, the patient is given high doses of toxic drugs to suppress the immune system, in turn making the patient more vulnerable to infection and disease. Isolating any illness from its relationship to the rest of the body like this runs completely against the holistic approach to health. The emphasis seems to be on relieving the obvious symptoms of the disorder, rather than on attempting to trace the wider imbalances that cause the problem.

Furthermore, general advice about the danger of a high cholesterol intake is given with little or no awareness of the way that fats really affect us. For example, we are often told to reduce the number of eggs we eat. Yet eggs are an invaluable source of many nutrients, and the fear that eggs cause a large buildup of blood cholesterol now appears to be largely unfounded. There is a limit to how much cholesterol can be absorbed in a single day and this is exceeded by a single egg. It seems apparent now that eggs do not adversely affect cholesterol levels; usually, the fat in our diets accounts for only 20 percent of the total cholesterol amount in the body. The rest is manufactured in the liver from carbohydrate.

Focusing on fat as the cause of heart disease is wrong. Instead we should look at the whole body and the metabolic pathways that affect fat and protein metabolism. When the body allows fat to accumulate—when your arteries harden and your blood pressure rises—it is a sign that these pathways are not working as they should. Amino acids and their cofactors are being used with increasing success to treat these heart problems. As the essential raw materials of your metabolic pathways, they work by repairing and rebalancing those damaged pathways which cause heart disease.

CRUCIAL PATHWAYS

The first pathway we'll look at involves using the amino acid methionine to relieve atherosclerosis. Put simply, a victim of atherosclerosis suffers from a buildup of fat in, and hardening of, the arteries. The subsequent rise in blood pressure and the intense stress this puts on the heart is one of the most common causes of eventual heart failure.

As the buildup of cholesterol and other fat products is one of the immediate causes of this hardening process, most doctors attribute atherosclerosis to the abundance of fatty foods in our diets. In fact, research conducted as long ago as 1906 identifies poor protein metabolism, rather than fat buildup, as the major cause, and in particular the blockage of a metabolic pathway involving methionine. In this pathway methionine is converted to the amino acid cystathione. At an intermediate stage of this cystathione-creating pathway, methionine becomes the amino acid homocysteine. This chemical is one of the causes of atherosclerosis.

In a normal, nutritionally balanced body, the entire pathway takes a split second to complete. Methionine becomes homocysteine, which in turn is instantly converted to cystathione. To convert homocysteine to cystathione, the body calls on an enzyme that is itself manufactured from a metabolic pathway involving several vitamins and amino acids. However, if any of the nutrients needed to manufacture this enzyme are missing, the conversion process is arrested, leaving homocysteine to circulate freely in the body.

But why is homocysteine so dangerous? Basically, because it's an abrasive. Passing through your bloodstream, it scratches and scrapes away at the delicate arterial walls like molecular sandpaper, causing the arteries to harden. In addition, the roughened areas it leaves also make ideal anchoring points for cholesterol and mineral deposits.

In time the arteries lose their pliability and clog up. The space available for the blood to flow shrinks. Simply to maintain the blood's normal circulating rate, blood pressure rises. The heart, pumping harder and more frequently, is working under severe stress, and its efficiency is reduced. Consequently, less oxygen reaches the cells. Frequent breathlessness, abnormal perspiration, and high heartbeat and pulse rate are common symptoms of this illness. Unless they are recognized in time, the victim may suffer a heart attack or a stroke.

Fortunately, by supplementing your diet with the specific amino acids and cofactors that convert methionine, all this can be avoided. The nutrients needed for the enzyme to complete the pathway are vitamin B_6 and the amino acid serine. B_6 is easily destroyed by heat; its levels in food drop sharply if cooked. When just this one substance is missing or depleted, the body simply won't be able to metabolize homocysteine to cystathione. But adding supplements of vitamin B_6 and serine to your diet provides your body with the materials it needs to make the enzyme and helps to lower the levels of homocysteine in the blood.

In a healthy body, homocysteine will also convert back to the parent molecule methionine. The substances the body requires to be able to do this include adequate amounts of existing methionine, several amino-based enzymes, and vitamin B_{12}.

Like B_6, B_{12} needs a special mention. It is a large molecule, and its absorption can take place only in a special section at the lower end of the small intestine. If you suffer from digestive disorders such as diarrhea, much of the B_{12} will simply pass straight through the body. To get through the intestinal wall, it also has to be coated with a mucinous protein called the "intrinsic factor," which itself depends on the presence of a variety of component amino acids. So even if you decide to take supplements of B_{12}, your digestion must be healthy in order to absorb them. The best way to ensure this is with a supplement of the complete amino acid blend, on top of the individual supplements. Easily absorbed, they help the pancreas manufacture all the necessary digestive enzymes.

You can see that deficiencies anywhere in the body cause problems far and wide. The complexity is amazing. Rather than thinking of atherosclerosis simply as the result of eating too much cholesterol, we must look at it as a symptom of complicated biochemical imbalances. It is the shock waves these imbalances send through the entire body that cause the condition. The way that amino acids and their cofactors can be used to relieve the condition shows the importance of a bodywide awareness of nutrition.

Fat Burn, Amino Style

Carnitine is another amino acid well worth including in any heart-relief formula. A deficiency of this amino allows fat to build up in the arteries, starves the cells of oxygen, and can lead to angina. Free-form carnitine supplements dredge the blood vessels of fat, which is then burned as bonus energy for your heart. All this leaves the heart able to perform more efficiently without subjecting it to undue stress.

Amino Heart Flush

Another highly beneficial amino acid is tryptophan. Research by a number of independent medical teams shows that regular dietary supplementation of just this one amino could prevent a staggering 15 percent of the deaths caused by heart attacks. Its effectiveness lies in the metabolic pathway that leads to the manufacture of serotonin. As well as helping us to sleep more soundly, the neuroinhibitory effects of this chemical also promote smoother, more regular muscle contractions throughout the body. This is important in preventing the heart spasms and racing heartbeat that often occur before a heart attack. It also helps to avoid the damage of fibrillation, which if left unchecked can lead to plaque buildup, hardening of the arteries, and raised blood pressure.

Including tryptophan in a blend with the other aminos we've looked at in this chapter helps to enhance the individual benefits of each of these supplements. Tryptophan and carnitine, for example, relieve the physical stresses on your heart—one by relaxing the muscle contraction, the other by feeding it more oxygen and energy. At the same time, methionine and serine, by getting rid of the abrasive homocysteine, make it easier for carnitine to flush the fat buildup from the artery walls.

One final amino to add to the blend is histidine. Its highly active form, histamine, is a calming neurotransmitter. It is also the most important substance released from the mast cells—the structures responsible for the reddening and flushing action of the immune system. This response is helpful in dealing with heart problems, as it forces more blood to the surface of the skin, lowers your overall blood pressure, and relieves the stresses on your heart. The niacin and nicotinic acid forms of B_3 also help to lower fat levels in the blood.

Earlier we referred to the image of a single falling pebble causing a landslide to explain how nutritional deficiency can lead to heart disease. Now imagine watching a film of this scene being played backward. Boulders seem to fly up the hill to relodge in their original places. The number of moving rocks gradually diminishes. Finally, we watch the pebble that started everything come to rest at the summit. Every stone is now back in its rightful place. This is the way that amino therapy works to relieve heart problems. Rather than conventional medicine, which would simply try to put the pebble back at the top without considering the destruction that has taken place, these amino supplements work by rectifying the entire landslide. In terms of your body, this means making sure that all the affected metabolic pathways are balanced and in harmony.

Let's look at a good heart-relief supplementation:

Aminos:
Methionine
Serine
Tryptophan
Histidine
Complete blend
Cofactors:
Vitamin B_3 (niacin or nicotinic acid)
Vitamin B_6
Vitamin B_{12}
Vitamin C
Vitamin E
Pantothenic acid
Folic acid

Magnesium
Zinc

This combination highlights the necessity of including vitamin and mineral cofactors. They are as important to the way your body uses amino acid supplements as cement is in keeping the bricks of your house in place.

Several notable researchers have shown that vitamin C is a key nutritional supplement in metabolizing cholesterol. Sherry Lewin, for example, found that sodium ascorbate (the mineral form of vitamin C) combines with molecules of an insoluble substance called calcium phospholipid, a compound formed from the minerals calcium and phosphorus, and excess cholesterol. Sticking to blood vessels like sludge, it can lead to atherosclerosis. This chemical is one of the fat by-products that carnitine and methionine help dislodge from the artery walls. Because it is insoluble, it continues to circulate in the blood until it finds another resting place; then it starts to accumulate all over again. However, when it meets with sodium ascorbate, they combine chemically to create calcium ascorbate and sodium phospholipid, both of which are soluble. The body then can easily eliminate the dangerous calcium phospholipid.

Vitamin C's ability to cleanse blood vessels is verified by Emil Getner. Experimenting with guinea pigs (one of those rare animals that, like human beings, are unable to produce vitamin C), he found that a shortage of vitamin C caused their veins and arteries to clog. When he administered high doses of vitamin C supplements, the blockages gradually cleared. Vitamin C, together with zinc, is also an important structural component of blood vessels, helping to maintain their ability to dilate.

Vitamin E, on the other hand, gives structural flexibility to red blood cells. This stops undue clotting, which in turn can lead to plaque buildup and eventual hemorrhaging. Vitamin E also prolongs the life of red blood cells and increases their oxygen-carrying capacity—immensely important in helping to reduce high blood pressure.

THE ESCAPE CLAWS

Another way of using amino acid supplements to treat heart problems is now receiving a lot of attention. This method is called chelation therapy. Chelation literally means "to form a claw." The process involves using special molecules to search the body like metabolic bloodhounds for dangerous and toxic minerals. When they find them, the searchers grasp them like claws, and the body is then able to eliminate the combined substances in the urine.

Of course, there are only a limited number of substances with structures that will chelate. The most effective are a small group of aminos headed by the versatile methionine. In addition to protecting blood vessels from fat buildup, methionine also acts as a chelator, guarding against calcium deposits. Excessive amounts of calcium in the walls of veins and arteries contribute to the hardening and fibrillation of the blood vessel walls called arteriosclerosis. Methionine supplements help to prevent this.

Chelators also work against free-radical activity. Much of the research into the effects of free-radical activity shows that the destruction they cause—ripping down cell membranes, oxidizing vitamins, and neutralizing vital enzymes—leads to the formation of atherones (fatty plaques). As these build up in the blood vessels, blood pressure rises and the heart and other organs are starved of oxygen. Doctors and nutritionists agree that heavy metals are major causes of heart disease and strokes, yet with the high levels of pollution in our cities, they seem unavoidable. Fortunately, by using amino acids to chelate these substances, we *can* avoid them.

In addition to methionine, the amino acid cysteine is an excellent chelator. Together with glycine and glutamic acid, cysteine is also part of glutathione. Glutathione is being used to chelate free radicals in a variety of illnesses, including allergies, rheumatism, and smoking complaints.

Finally, some experts are starting to use the amino acid ethylene diametetranetic acid (EDTA), which is one of the most powerful chelators known. The problem with EDTA, which arises to a lesser extent with all chelators, is that it isn't selective about which minerals it claws on to. An example of this is the way that EDTA is used commercially in the food-processing industry. Scalding vegetables such as broccoli, peas, and spinach with EDTA removes all heavy metals from their surfaces so that they appear lustrously green, rather than their natural grayer appearance. But when these vegetables are analyzed, not only are the levels of heavy metals like lead or chromium lower, but nutritious substances like zinc and manganese are also found to be depleted to about 20 percent of their normal levels. The same thing may happen with chelation therapy in the body. It's important to seek advice from a qualified doctor or nutritionist before using EDTA. He or she will monitor the mineral levels in your body and recommend specific nutrients should their levels drop.

So how do the supplements mentioned in this chapter work in practice? Let's find out by looking at a case history. Rob is a warehouse laborer in his midforties. His physically demanding job involves shifting crates that weigh up to a hundred pounds. He has never smoked, hardly drinks, and is active in his spare time as well as at work. One day, unloading a truck, he felt a sharp, stabbing pain in his chest and a dull sensation in his legs, almost as if they had gone to sleep. Hospital tests showed that his arteries were severely hardened and clogged. "The doctor said it was only because I was so strong and active that I hadn't had a heart attack," Rob said. Unfortunately there was nothing the doctor could do to reverse the clogging process. He put Rob on a course of drugs designed to keep the symptoms at bay and told him to reduce his exertion at work. He was to come back in six months for a checkup, when they would decide whether a bypass operation was needed.

During the following months, Rob's wife Michelle read about the benefits of amino testing and therapy. Anxious to try anything that might help him, she made an appointment for her husband to come for nutritional counseling. After the usual tests, he was first recommended the complete amino blend to stimulate the enzyme systems throughout his body. In addition, he was told to take a blend of the three aminos that form the chelator glutathione (cysteine, glutamic acid, and glycine), as well as carnitine and methionine. The cofactors included vitamin B_6, vitamin B complex, magnesium, manganese, zinc, and sodium ascorbate (the mineral vitamin C). A few weeks later, Michelle telephoned. "Rob suddenly has so much energy," she said. "Is it all right if I take the formulation, too? I won't be able to keep up with him otherwise."

At the end of the six months, Rob returned to his doctor for the checkup. "He was so surprised," Rob recalled, "for a moment he thought he'd mixed up his case notes, because my arteries were in such great shape. He said, 'I don't know what you've been doing, but keep it up.' "

17

An End to
Digestive Troubles

Digestion is a crucial part of the body's metabolic equation. It is the balance between the food you eat and the use your body makes of it. Suffering from poor digestion upsets this balance and causes your body more harm than you probably imagine. You may eat an excellent diet, with a full balance of all the vitamins, minerals, and proteins you need. But unless the food is digested properly, your body simply won't be able to grow and repair itself as it should.

We've all suffered from an upset or acid stomach. Most of us have probably embarrassed ourselves in company with an accidental burp or wind. Usually these occurrences are merely symptoms of a mildly unsettled intestinal tract. Occasionally, though, they may signify that something is giving your digestion serious trouble. If you smoke, for example, the chances are high that you suffer from depleted stomach acids and enzyme levels. Constipation and/or diarrhea often result from allergies. The stress of emotional difficulties can lead to ulcers and colitis. Even the quality of the food itself is often to blame for your problems.

Whatever the cause, the simple fact is that when your

digestion doesn't work as it should, your cells are starved of the nutrients they need for healthy living. Toxins that cause oxidation and cell degeneration are allowed to build up. Growth and resistance to disease are reduced. Your skin gets blotchy; your body feels heavier and more sluggish; your emotions become exaggerated and unstable. Remember, your digestive system is a pipeline carrying vital nutrients from the food to your cells. Bad digestion cuts off that pipeline.

Amino acids could have been invented for these problems. When they are in their free-form state, separated from the long protein molecule chains, the body doesn't need the intestinal tract to break them down. For all intents and purposes, they are predigested. They pass quickly and easily through the intestinal wall into the bloodstream. And from there they can help to reestablish normal digestive functions, strengthening the pancreas and stimulating the production of digestive acids and enzymes. This chapter will follow your food on its passage through the gastrointestinal system. Then, seeing where and how problems arise, we can prescribe amino formulas that will help to restore the delicate digestive balance between your food and your body.

ACID REMARKS

In the food-rich West, we overeat. The opportunities for overindulgence, not to say gluttony, are everywhere: on holidays, at parties, in restaurants, and on the overflowing shelves of supermarkets. The problem with this abundance is that many people simply do not have enough stomach acid to cope with it. In their book, *Psychodietetics*, Drs. Cheraskin and Ringsdorff record their examination of over three thousand victims of gastrointestinal disorders. They found that the problems of a third of this group stemmed simply from insufficient stomach acid.

Stomach acid is important because it is the first stage of digestion. Any problems here will be magnified enormously by the time the food passes into your intestines. Let's see why.

Usually, when it reaches the stomach, your food activates the release of hydrochloric acid. This acid environment is important for stimulating the enzyme pepsin into action. Pepsin digests approximately 15 percent of the food before it passes on to the small intestine. But for those people who suffer from low stomach acid—caused perhaps by smoking, heavy drinking, or even as part of the natural process of aging—the percentage will be much less.

One of the first results of this drop in stomach acid is that the food will literally start to ferment. Here's why: Your body permits the growth of a certain amount of bacteria and yeast to aid digestion. As we discovered in Chapter 14, the threat of any dangerous expansion of the intestine's yeast colony is kept in check by acids and enzymes. Stresses inhibit enzyme production and allow the yeast to flourish. Insufficient acid, leading to low pepsin levels, is one such stress. It lets the yeast colony become so metabolically overactive that it causes fermentation. Large quantities of carbohydrate are turned into alcohol. In some cases, this is so serious that victims literally get drunk on the carbohydrates they eat. It distorts consciousness, puts massive stress on their liver and kidneys, and often leads to obesity and hypoglycemia. Like alcoholics needing a drink, they simply cannot live without eating increasing amounts of carbohydrate food.

Few people realize that this can be traced back to a yeast problem in the intestines—still fewer that low stomach acid levels are directly responsible. We estimate that as many as nine out of ten stomach upsets mistakenly attributed to acid indigestion—too much acid in the stomach—are actually the result of yeast fermentation from too *little* acid. The common response? Reach for the antacid tablets, of course. But this only serves to reduce acid levels still further and is the worst thing you can do.

The consequences of low stomach acid don't end here.

Worse is to come as the undigested, fermenting food reaches the small intestine. This is where the body secretes digestive enzymes—a different one for each amino acid link of the protein chain in an ideal body, at least. But with your body already under the stresses caused by depleted stomach acid, the pancreas can't cope with the increased quantity of undigested food. Much of the food, therefore, just sits in the intestines and putrefies, releasing potentially harmful substances. The results of this may range from subtle changes of behavior—how well you remember and think—to severe emotional problems like anxiety, depression, and even schizophrenia. In time this leads to diarrhea, even chronic diarrhea. Putrid-smelling flatulence and feces, and a powerful, unpleasant body odor, are common physical symptoms of putrefaction.

Remember, all the problems we've looked at so far stem from depleted stomach acid. And the implications of this depletion go beyond even these serious health problems. Look at this quote from Newbold's *Vitamin C Against Cancer*: "I have found . . . that [cancer] patients are either hypo- or achlohydric [have little or no stomach acid]. In order for them to get any nutrition you've got to supplement their stomach acid."

The first thing to do, then, is to raise the stomach acid levels in your stomach to allow digestion to take place. Free-form, "predigested," amino acids do not require any stomach acid and act to help raise stomach acid. The body will absorb them, even though the acid and enzyme levels are low. Furthermore, many experts believe that because individual free-form aminos are not complete foods in themselves, they won't be attacked by the ravenous bacterial population.

So which aminos are the most helpful?

First, we recommend a supplement containing the complete amino blend (see Chapter 7). As almost every enzyme depends on amino acids for its structure, when digestion is inefficient, your body is robbed of the nutrients it needs to create these enzymes. The complete amino blend contains the nutrients the body needs to manufacture its enzymes from scratch. This blend—the master protector against illness—also helps rid the body of many of the ill effects of poor digestion. Many of the amino acids in the complete blend provide nutritional first aid to cells depleted by poor digestion. Aminos like carnitine and glutathionine clear blood vessels of toxins and fats. And phenylalanine, tyrosine, and methionine help to improve your emotional stability and mental alertness.

Then, to help raise your acid levels, your diet should include additional amounts of glutamic acid HCL, histidine, and glycine. Glutamic acid HCL is a widely available free-form amino supplement mixed with hydrochloric acid (HCL). Providing hydrochloric acid this way is the quickest and most direct method of raising the stomach acid levels to help digestion. Glutamic acid itself has several important digestive functions. For people with high carbohydrate intake and fermentation in the intestines, it helps to regulate blood sugar levels. This eases the stress on the insulin-producing pancreas, allowing it instead to secrete the necessary digestive enzymes into the small intestine.

Glutamine, the form of glutamic acid lacking a hydrogen atom, has been found to help decrease alcohol consumption by working on the appetite centers in the hypothalamus. In this way, your carbohydrate dependency can be reduced, in turn cutting down the degree of carbohydrate fermentation in the stomach and small intestine.

What about the two remaining digestion-helping aminos on our list, histidine and glycine? In the stomach—as opposed to the intestines—histamine (a product of histidine) promotes natural secretions of stomach acid. It also increases the amount of saliva in the mouth. Glycine, too, has been found to improve acid secretion. Here's an acid-stimulating blend you might try:

Aminos:
Glutamic acid HCL
Histidine
Glycine

Cofactors:
Vitamin B_3
Vitamin B_6
Vitamin C as ascorbic acid
Betaine HCL (Widely available as a dry acid supplement.
    It is not an amino itself which is why it is included as a
    cofactor.)

The value of these amino acid supplements simply cannot be overstated. A good analogy is to examine the
sprinter's starting blocks at a track meet. In a race, where
the margin of victory is measured in hundredths of a
second, the blocks must be set perfectly to give a sprinter the
maximum possible impetus when pushing off. If they are
wrongly spaced—or if the sprinter starts without any blocks
at all—he or she might be the fastest alive, but in the effort
to catch up with the other competitors, he or she will
overstride, lose natural rhythm, and come in last. Stomach
acid is your digestive starting block. As the food you eat is
only as good as the way it is digested, this amino acid
formula will give it precisely the start it needs.

MORE PROBLEMS
FURTHER DOWN

Not all digestive problems stem from low-stomach acid and
enzyme levels. An increasingly common problem in our age
of refined food is the lack of fiber in our diets. Fiber is the
indigestible part of the food which helps the muscle
contractions of the intestinal wall—peristalsis—to draw it
through the alimentary canal. The time it takes normal,
high-fiber food to pass through the body is between 24 and
48 hours. The less fiber you have in your diet, though, the
longer it will take. Many people suffer from transit times of
four days or more.

This is itself a cause of serious intestinal disorders. First,
as they move so slowly, the feces lose water through the
intestinal wall, becoming harder and more rasping in the

process. The greater physical friction of the passing food causes small pouches to form on the intestinal wall. These pouches—called diverticulosis—only serve to slow the food even further. The longer the food remains in the intestines, the more damage the toxic by-products will do. They can cause anything from varicose veins to appendicitis to cancer of the colon. Also, undigested protein starts to leak through the intestinal wall, causing allergic reactions. If you often feel bloated and sluggish, even a long time after eating, excrete hard stools, and suffer from headaches and unaccountable joint pains, this could be your problem.

But these physical symptoms aren't all. In the large intestine, the diverticulosis pouches often become inflamed: this is called diverticulitis. It can lead to the discomfort and suffering of ulcers, rectal bleeding, and hemorrhoids. In addition to the physical pain, many psychologists now recognize a connection between this and severe mental disturbances. Accumulating in the pouches, often over many years, the bacteria and toxic by-products may be responsible for abnormal anxiety, tension, manic-depression, and perhaps even schizophrenia. It is almost unheard of for colitis sufferers to be unaffected by these problems. Traditionally, doctors believed that stress could affect intestinal disorders by slowing down digestive functions—but not vice versa. It now seems probable that intestinal problems are just as likely to cause stress. Each effectively helps perpetuate the other.

Recognizing the link between the two, many experts find that one of the best forms of treatment is the amino anxiety formula—tryptophan, histidine, taurine, and glycine.

Tryptophan and histidine act as powerful neuroinhibitors. Extra histamine increases the calming alpha wave activity of your brain. These brain waves help your body's parasympathetic nervous system to operate effectively. This is the side of your autonomic nervous system that is responsible for digestive functions—for pumping blood to the intestines and stimulating peristalsis. Additional histidine, therefore, helps the intestines to digest your food more efficiently. Tryptophan, as the precursor of serotonin, also soothes your mental activity. So when stress does occur, it lets your body cope with it a lot more effectively. This ensures that blood needed for digestion will stay in the intestines rather than being diverted to the heavy muscles as part of the stress response. It also allows enzyme secretion to continue normally.

Unlike histidine and tryptophan, which work in the brain, glycine and taurine inhibit the excitory actions of the central nervous system. This has the effect of relaxing the bowel muscles, allowing smoother peristaltic contractions and quicker transit times.

Taken before your high-fiber meal, the anxiety formula is invaluable in helping your body get the full nutritional benefit from its food. Then, once the food is digested, this formula ensures that the waste products will be ejected smoothly and quickly, preventing a harmful buildup of toxins.

Here is the high-anxiety blend. It should be taken at least an hour before a high-fiber meal:

Aminos:
Tryptophan
Histidine
Glycine
Taurine
Cofactors:
Vitamin B_1
Vitamin B_2
Vitamin B_6
Vitamin C
Calcium
Zinc

Note: *Don't forget to consult Chapter 5, "Safety and Precautions" to ensure that you can take this blend safely.*

Philip is a mountaineer in his late thirties, leading an active and vigorous life in Scotland. "I've always been very moody," he said, "I used to like putting it down to a 'volatile Celtic temperament.' The trouble was that last year I went from the occasionally irritable to the downright unstable. I started going through fits of bottomless, black depression. Any mental effort seemed to be too much. I remember once bursting into tears when I couldn't think of a word I wanted to use in an article I was writing. At the same time, my body lost its vitality. I could hardly walk upstairs without my legs feeling like lead, let alone walk up a mountain." His dismay deepened when he noticed that varicose veins had appeared on his calves. Furthermore, during this period—about eight months—he gained nearly 14 pounds.

Describing these and other symptoms—stiff joints, a craving for sweets and cakes, and painfully hard stools—it was clear that Philip was suffering from chronic digestive difficulties. He was prescribed the complete amino digestive program: the anxiety formula (pages 108-9), together with phenylalanine, betaine HCL (the dry acid supplement), and glutamic acid HCL, both to provide the body with extra acid and to satisfy his carbohydrate craving—all supplementing a diet high in fiber.

Within three weeks his body felt mentally and physically clearer than it ever had in his life. "I realized all that stuff about the dour Celtic moodiness was rubbish," he admitted. "It was as if I'd been viewing my life through a dirty windshield. Now that it's clean, I can't believe how I ever managed before. As for my body, it feels lighter, more resilient, and I have to walk twice as far to burn up all the energy."

Constipation

As well as amino acids, fiber was important in helping Philip recover. A few words of warning, though: When you decide on a high-fiber diet to accompany the amino formulas, beware of the pitfalls. Many people mistakenly think that bran will satisfy all their fiber needs. In fact, wheat bran can be quite harmful. Its scraping action often irritates an already inflamed bowel. When this happens the intestinal wall secretes mucus to protect itself. This has the effect of making the food pass rapidly through the body to give the bowel a chance to heal itself. If the bemused victim of constipation suddenly finds himself suffering from diarrhea, this could be the cause. Bran also decreases the absorption of important minerals like magnesium, calcium, and zinc. Instead of bran, try increasing your consumption of other natural fiber sources such as grains, fresh fruit, and vegetables. Their colon-cleansing action is far better than bran. After all, which would you use on your car, a chamois cloth or a brillo pad? These nonirritating bran sources will also help regulate your blood sugar levels.

Chronic Diarrhea

For most people, diarrhea is unpleasant but short-lived. Some, however, as a result perhaps of an allergy or an irritated bowel, suffer chronically. It is a deceptively dangerous problem as it prevents the victims from getting any benefit from their food at all—the intestinal wall simply has no time to absorb the nutrients. This is known as chronic diarrhea, and if it is allowed to continue it can lead to severe malnourishment. Sufferers are often thin, finding it impossible to put on any weight, however much they eat. In the case of young children, it can be particularly serious, as it might halt their growth altogether. Happily, chronic diarrhea responds particularly well to high doses of the complete amino blend (see page 62). In the early stages of recovery, the victim's intestinal tract is often so sensitive that amino acids and their cofactors—having no bulk or fiber—are the only substances it will tolerate.

18
Allergy Answers

Most people are only dimly aware of how allergies affect them. Some know from experience to dread the start of summer and the inevitable attack of hay fever—with its months of headaches, watery eyes, and stuffy noses. Others are reluctant to visit friends with pets because they are allergic to cat or dog fur. Beyond these common examples, though, general knowledge and understanding of allergies is almost nonexistent.

Yet in reality people are allergic to an enormous variety of substances. Tobacco smoke, for example, causes a reaction in almost everybody; many people can't drink milk or eat wheat without becoming ill; and numerous pollutants and chemicals affect us continually—all without us realizing. How often do you have a "low day," physically drained and mentally sluggish, unable to eat without feeling queasy, perhaps with trouble breathing? What about the sores and ulcers in your mouth? Or the rash of dry, flaky skin on the backs of your arms? These are all symptoms of allergies. In fact, if you suffer from rheumatoid arthritis, there is a good chance that this, too, is caused by an allergy.

An allergy is an abnormally heightened sensitivity to a substance (allergen) that is brought into contact with the body. The traditional view that this sensitivity can be traced back to a single cause, and steps taken to either avoid it or "desensitize" your body to it, is obsolete. There is such an incredible number of allergens that in many people allergic reactions occur continually. A radical new approach is needed—one that strengthens the body's entire metabolism, and in doing so mitigates its allergy-causing hypersensitivity. Over the past few years, amino acids have been used in this way with astonishing success. They attack the causes of allergies at their roots. By improving your digestion, removing damage-causing agents such as free radicals, and balancing the resources of your body's immune system, they offer hope for literally millions of allergy sufferers.

THE HIDDEN ALLERGY: PROTEIN

The first allergy we'll look at is caused by the body's sensitivity to undigested protein. The protein we eat must be broken down in the intestines before being absorbed. Occasionally, however, protein chains manage to seep through the intestinal wall intact. The allergic response this causes—reddening, swelling, and flushing of the skin, for instance—occurs when the protein comes into contact with highly sensitive tissue hormones called kinins. The kinins respond by tearing down the walls of neighboring mast cells to release the substances contained inside: histamine, serotonin, and heparin. Histamine, in particular, creates symptoms that range from mild fatigue, watery eyes, and blocked-up nose to painful, suppurating rashes and aching muscles. It may lower your blood pressure, restrict the movement of blood, or cause slower muscle contractions. Sore back muscles and the difficulty that asthmatics have in inhaling are often caused by this constrictive process.

The inflammation that mast cells cause can be particu-

larly harmful if it happens around the nerves. Kinin
inflammation can even affect the brain, leading to headaches, migraine, nausea, and lethargy. In extreme cases,
experts have found that it will even cause schizophrenia.

Remember, these are all symptoms of the body's allergy
to foreign proteins, and the cause lies in the simple inability of many people to digest their food. Without adequate
levels of digestive enzymes to break the protein chains down
into their constituent amino acids, the protein chains either
sit in the intestines and putrefy or begin to seep through the
intestinal wall. Once this happens, they are quickly absorbed into the blood. The blood's circulatory system
distributes food so efficiently that the offending proteins
that escape from the intestines will soon come into contact
with the kinins, reacting almost anywhere in the body. As
well as the kinin and mast cell reactions, the intestinal wall
itself often responds to contact with these renegade proteins
by secreting an extra layer of mucus to protect itself. This
has a lubricating effect and often leads to diarrhea.

When their sinuses start hurting, or when they suffer an
asthma attack, few people imagine that the blame might lie
with their digestion. Instead they try to relieve the symptoms by taking a synthetic antidepressant or an anti-
inflammatory synthetic hormone. Sometimes they might
turn to plain and simple aspirin. Yet the side effects of these
substances are often worse than the disorder.

Rather than suppress these allergy symptoms (which is
what conventional drug therapy does best), amino acids
work by attacking the *causes* of the allergies. Let's see what
kind of formula you can use to prevent protein seepage.
First, if your stomach acid levels need raising, you can
include supplements of glutamic acid HCl and histidine in
your diet. The ability of these aminos to stimulate stomach
acid release and raise the levels of pepsin—the stomach
enzyme—has been proved many times in the last decade.
Glutamic acid also helps ease the stresses on the pancreas,
the gland that manufactures all the digestive enzymes. Two
enzymes are especially important—chymotrypsin and car-

boxypeptase—because they reduce inflammation caused by the kinins. However, every enzyme is vital for thorough digestion. To ensure that the pancreas has all the necessary raw materials for its job, you should also include in your formula a supplement of the complete amino acid blend. Finally, to raise you from allergy-induced torpor, take phenylalanine. As the precursor of adrenalin and noradrenalin, it helps to stimulate you physically and mentally. So your protection against protein peptides should include:

Aminos:
Complete blend
Glutamic acid HCl
Histidine
Phenylalanine
Cofactors:
Vitamin B_3
Vitamin B_6
Vitamin C

MECHANICS OF IMMUNITY

Of course, if undigested protein were the only cause of allergies, life would be much easier than it is. In fact, the number of allergens is almost unlimited. It includes drugs, pollen and molds, animal fur, dandruff, bacteria, many different foods, smoke, and pollution. Depending on how the allergens contact the body—either by ingestion in the intestines or the lungs, or absorption through the skin—they may cause fever, rashes, diarrhea, headaches, or arthritis. The only characteristic that all allergens have in common is the abnormal, hypersensitive reaction they cause.

At the root of this response is the thymus gland, which guards against invaders such as virus infections by secreting a hormone called thymosin. This hormone orders the spleen and the lymph nodes to produce defenses against the invaders: T-cells and B-cells.

B-cells, also known as antibodies, are amino acid structures that unite with the invading allergen to render it harmless. If the allergen is a toxin, the antibody neutralizes it. If it is bacteria, the antibody coats it like a second skin, insulating it from the threatened tissue. If the allergen happens to be a virus, the antibody blocks the attachment points between it and the cell it is trying to infect. Collectively, antibodies are called the immunoglobins (Ig), and this grouping is split into five subgroups—A, D, E, G, and M.

Each group performs a different role in the immune system. All the IgM antibodies, for example, are responsible for neutralizing toxins. Because of the way their connecting sites (the area on the surface of the antibody that makes contact with the invader) are structured, antibodies are selective, but not quite exclusive, about what they attack.

Now let's look at the other branch of the immune system, the T-cells. These are divided into several groups—lymphocytes, lymphokines, and macrophages, as well as helper and suppressor cells. Lymphokines, the body's natural drugs, cause the rashes that result from contact with allergens such as poison ivy. T-cells also cooperate with B-cell antibodies. When T-cells meet an invader, the number of helper cells compared to suppressor cells increases. This in turn raises the number of antibodies present to fight the allergen. Conversely, suppressor cells literally suppress the rate of antibody production. So the number of circulating T-cells in the overall total isn't the only important figure; the balance between helpers and suppressors matters as well. If the number of helpers constantly outweighs the suppressors, your immune system will become oversensitive, and allergic reactions will start to occur.

WHEN ALLERGIES FLARE UP

Most allergies can be traced back to two related sources. The first is that the immune systems of as many as one person in ten produce more T-cell helpers than suppressors. These helper cells lead to the formation of increased numbers of antibodies, even though there may be no dangerous invading substances in the body. If these antibodies reacted exclusively to the substances they were designed to fight, this overproduction would be harmless. But, because invading substances change—viruses, for example, are constantly altering their structures—the defending antibodies must also be able to adapt in order to be effective. For this to happen, the structures of their connecting sites allow for a certain latitude in what they latch on to. So when their numbers are abnormally increased by T-cell helpers, and in the absence of any harmful substances for them to attack, the antibodies might turn on almost anything as an invader. The result will be the symptoms of an immune response—headache, inflammation, fever—as the antibodies start reacting to the most innocuous, everyday substances: dust, pollen, foods, and even the body's own tissue.

The second related cause of this allergy response is the IgE group of antibodies. As its main purpose is to fight parasitic diseases, IgE has become almost unnecessary in developed countries. During an abnormal increase in T-cell helpers, IgE fixes itself to the histamine-containing mast cells. When it encounters an allergen, it breaks open the cell wall, spilling the contents. This produces the familiar symptoms of sneezing, runny nose, and inflammation that we've already looked at.

So how can we use amino acids to treat these antibody responses? One of the most effective forms of allergy relief is supplemental histidine. Not only does histidine stimulate stomach acid secretion, it also regulates the ratio of helper cell to suppressor. This is a little surprising, as its histimine form is a central component of the allergy response—the flushing and inflammation. Histidine's suppressor-helper balancing action actively prevents this allergic response from occurring. Histidine supplementation can unblock nasal passages, resolve redness and swelling, and relieve the irritability, depression, and anxiety that often accompany an allergy response. When it comes to mitigating allergic responses, histidine is one of the best aminos you can take.

When Steven, a bookseller, first came for nutritional counseling, he was suffering from hay fever—although he looked more like the losing contender of a boxing match. His eyes were as swollen as lemons; his nose was a livid mauve, streaming constantly; and he spoke with a slurred, asthmatic wheeze. Rather than carrying out the usual tests, we advised him to take supplemental histidine three times a day for an initial two weeks, before deciding on a fuller course of treatment. Steven telephoned less than a week later to say that he wouldn't be visiting again, as his symptoms had completely disappeared. Listening to him speak, in a voice that gave no hint of asthma or inflammation, it was hard to believe he was the same person.

FREE RADICALS: BIOLOGICAL PIRATES

What is it that initially causes the body to create more helper cells than suppressors, and how can we remedy it? For the answer let's pay a visit to the free radicals. Free radicals are one of the greatest threats to health. Excessive levels of heavy metals in the air or your food lead to the creation of free radicals. Radiation and ultraviolet light create free radicals, as does any sort of illness or injury to tissue.

A free radical's only goal in life is to find another electron to balance its atomic charge. It will stop at nothing to get it. Plundering the protein structures of your body in its search, it oxidizes cells, causing inflammation, injury, and destruction. And it raises the toxicity levels in your body, placing the immune system under greater stress.

Free-radical activity in fats creates dangerous peroxides. You can tell this yourself by smelling butter that has been left for too long and has become rancid. Free-radical-generated rancidity also occurs in the essential unsaturated fatty acids of your body and is one of the major causes of increased helper cell activity.

Basically, the peroxides that result from free-radical activity work as blocking agents. They prevent a substance in the fatty acids from metabolizing to a short-lived regulating molecule called prostoglandin El (PGEl). It is PGEl that stimulates the function of the T-cell suppressors. Without it the T-cell ratio is disrupted, and, as we've seen, the body becomes hypersensitive to a variety of harmless substances.

PGEl is converted in four stages from a component in the essential fatty acids called linoleic acid. The first stage of the transformation pathway converts linoleic acid to gamma-linoleic acid, and it is this conversion that the free radicals prevent. This can lead not only to common food allergies and a sensitivity to fur and pollen, but also to autoimmune diseases such as rheumatoid arthritis.

How can we protect ourselves from free-radical damage? One answer is with glutathione.

Glutathione is a tripeptide. This means that it's made from three amino acids: cysteine, glutamic acid, and glycine. In the body, glutathione combines with the mineral selenium to produce an enzyme called glutathione peroxidase synthase. Tests have shown that using glutathione to increase the levels of this enzyme in the body prove remarkably successful in helping to relieve allergic responses. Acting as a free-radical scavenger, glutathione peroxidase synthase helps prevent the formation of fatty acid peroxides. This, in turn, allows the metabolism of PGEl to occur normally.

Since it works on all autoimmune illnesses, glutathione can reduce the inflammation, tissue degeneration, and pain of rheumatoid arthritis. It is also an excellent chelator, removing from the body dangerous accumulations of heavy metals such as cadmium and lead—themselves sources of free radicals. It is even being used experimentally to clear up sources of airborne pollutants—such as factory smoke, chemicals, and bacteria—from lung tissue. All these substances are major causes of allergies. Before long, we might be using glutathione to treat allergies caused by anything from car fumes to pollen, milk, and even the gluten in wheat.

As glutathione is a tripeptide, taking it as a complete supplement means that much of it might be broken down by the proteolytic enzymes in the intestines. Also, glutathione is expensive. So instead of taking it in a complete dose, many people prefer to take a blend of its three constituent aminos, together with selenium, since these aminos act as a base from which your body can manufacture glutathione. A good blend for glutathione should include:

Aminos:
Histidine
Glycine
Cysteine
Glutamic acid
Cofactors:
Selenium
Vitamin B
Vitamin C

Allergies are one of today's major health problems. Some experts in the field even insist that every single illness, from arthritis to cancer, is allergy-related. Whether this is true or not, much of the conventional allergy therapy has tended to treat the obvious symptoms, rather than attempt to come to grips with the deeper causes. Even some of the most respected forms of therapy currently available deal only with individual allergies, instead of questioning why a patient should be allergic to particular substances in the first place. Now, thanks to amino-based nutritional therapy, we can truly start to combat the fundamental causes of allergy.

19
Sex and Amino Acids

When sex works for us, it can make us feel rich emotionally and physically. It also brings us closer to our partner and makes us more loving. Unfortunately, it doesn't work for everyone. Sexual problems, in one form or another, are widespread and can be a source of intense suffering and anxiety. For those who have experienced frigidity, impotence, and other difficulties, sex has become a source of frustration, anger, and resentment—making them feel unjustly imprisoned in a body devoid of passion.

Fulfillment depends on more than emotional factors. For sex to work, things have to be right biochemically. This is where amino acids can be helpful. For by strengthening the relevant metabolic pathways, it is possible to banish impotence, cure frigidity, and even stimulate fertility, providing real hopes of conception for many childless couples.

IN SEARCH OF ORGASM

Perhaps the most widespread sexual problem today is the difficulty many women have in achieving orgasm. Until now, nonorgasmic women have been given psychotherapy, often without results. Even the unkind, almost rebuking term that describes this condition, *frigidity*, suggests a mental attitude in the sufferer—an offhandedness or lack of passion—rather than a physical inability.

Recently, however, research has shown that frigidity is often physiological in origin. It can be corrected by supplementing the diet with a combination of specific free-form amino acids such as lysine, arginine, and histidine. Of these, the most important free-form amino is histidine.

Histidine needs to be present in good quantity for orgasm to take place. This amino acid is the parent of the active molecule histamine. Orgasm is triggered when histamine is released in the body from the mast cells in the genitals. These cells function as part of the immune system, but also cause the sexual flush experienced during arousal. For both functions, the active ingredient is histamine. When there is insufficient histidine in the body, histamine production is low and women find it difficult, sometimes even impossible, to achieve orgasm. The result is frigidity, with its destructive by-products of guilt and anger.

Histamine's effects on orgasm have been well-documented for over a decade by the American researcher Carl Pfeiffer. He conducted a study on frigid women and discovered that, although most of his subjects suffered from low levels of many of the amino acids, their histamine levels were particularly low. He reasoned that if these women took extra histidine, they might experience orgasm for the first time. It worked. Without any psychotherapy, the women who had been given histidine broke the bonds of frigidity, achieving an enormous sense of liberation.

Since then histidine has often been used in this way by sophisticated nutritional counselors. It is either given in the form of a 500-mg dose before each meal, or as part of a larger and better-balanced sex formula, which we will look at more closely at the end of the chapter.

To achieve orgasm, a woman might try these nutrients taken before each meal:

Aminos:
Histidine
Lysine
Arginine
Cofactors:
Vitamin B_3
Vitamin B_6
Manganese

TOO MUCH, TOO SOON

Pfeiffer also examined the benefit of histidine for men, discovering what a two-edged sword it is. Male orgasm is a localized reflex caused by the release of histamine from a large concentration of mast cells in the penis head. As expected, the circulating levels of histidine played a significant role, both in the ability of a man to climax and in the time it takes him. The higher the levels, the shorter the time needed—so much so that for a few this led to another problem: premature ejaculation.

Pfeiffer then extended his studies to men suffering from premature ejaculation. He discovered that their high histamine levels could be lowered by methionine, taken with a little calcium as a cofactor. These men are now able to lead more satisfying sex lives.

How does it all work? Rather than directly competing with histidine, the methionine is converted into its active form, s-adenosyl-methionine, a substance that is needed to help create adrenalin. Adrenalin is a most important chemical in controlling the body's sexual activity—it mitigates the effects of high histamine levels, and so delays orgasm.

To prevent premature ejaculation, try this formula:
Amino:
Methionine
Cofactor:
Calcium
Magnesium

AMINO KEYS TO FERTILITY

But good sex is not always an end in itself. At some point most people want children. Yet for many, these hopes go tragically unfulfilled. These couples feel disappointed and frustrated. For a few—those who see having children as the *raison d'etre* of their relationship—it can even threaten a breakup. Even in the most balanced and open of relationships, infertility may create enormous strains.

Increasing Sperm Count

A major cause of this problem lies in low sperm count. In recent years, the average sperm count of men in the West has decreased dramatically. No one knows why. Some scientists attribute it to the cumulative polluting and poisoning of the planet. Others see the additives we use to process our foods, or the hormones fed to livestock, as responsible. Whatever the cause, the fact is that the average male sperm count has declined from 100 million per cubic centimeter at the turn of the century to less than 25 million today—dangerously close to the level of sterility. Too many men have now fallen beneath it.

Amino acids can come to the rescue here as well. As long ago as 1926, research into the composition of semen revealed the presence of two chemicals that we now call spermidine and spermine. But it wasn't until the mid-1960s that they were found to play a major role in the synthesis of semen. It is these two amino acids which give semen its characteristic odor. More important, tests carried out on vasectomy patients and women using the contraceptive pill (two groups that, like men suffering from low sperm count, have undergone a loss of fertility) showed much lower concentrations of these two amino acids than people outside these groups. It was therefore logical for biochemists to assume that supplements of the amino acid parent molecule of spermidine and spermine, given to men suffering from low sperm count, would ease their problems. And indeed it has.

The parent amino acid of spermine is arginine. In one recent study, 42 men suffering from low sperm count were given arginine together with its cofactors. Each patient showed an almost 100 percent increase in his sperm count shortly after the trials began. Better still, the motility—the ability of the individual sperm to move—was also greatly increased. This is important if the sperm is to reach the egg so that fertilization can occur. When researchers withdrew the arginine, the sperm count immediately dropped. It rose again when the amino acid was readministered. As a remedy for low sperm production, try these nutrients:

Aminos:
Arginine
Methionine
Cofactors:
Manganese
Vitamin B_6

Fertility Nutrition

Even if a man's sperm count has been successfully raised, his partner might still be unable to conceive, often because of undetected nutritional deficiencies. If this is the case, amino acid supplements can also greatly increase her chances of conception.

A successful pregnancy needs the support of two important hormones: follicle-stimulating hormone (FSH), which is mainly responsible for the growth and development of the ovaries, and leutenizing hormone (LH), whose chief function is to promote ovulation. Both these hormones contain long chains of amino acids. Of course, a full and balanced supply of all the essential amino acids is vital in the formation of the hormone molecules. The cysteine content in these two hormones is particularly high, so this amino is especially important.

In addition to cysteine, vitamin C helps the replenishment of the ovaries (especially when their growth is being stimulated by the action of FSH), and vitamin E is important for the maintenance of the cell membrane of the sex organs.

A nutritional program for female infertility needs to be carefully tailored to a woman's individual needs. However, most programs are based around a daily balance of nutrients that looks like this:

Aminos:
Arginine
Cysteine
Histidine
Methionine
Phenylalanine
Cofactors:
Vitamin B_3
Vitamin B_6
Vitamin E
Vitamin C
Folic acid
Zinc
Selenium
Magnesium

PRENATAL HELP

Even after conceiving, some women find themselves faced with the threat of a miscarriage. The most important hormone during pregnancy is progesterone. To put it simply, if progesterone is deficient, the pregnancy will end prematurely. On the other hand, too much progesterone will extend pregnancy beyond its natural span.

Unlike FHS and LH, progesterone is not an amino acid structure. The most important molecule in this pathway is cholesterol. Pregnant women mustn't try to avoid it in their diets. In this area, too, metabolic nutrition based on free-form amino acids can be enormously helpful. A daily formula for helping to maintain pregnancy might look like this:

Aminos:
Glutamine
Tyrosine
Lysine

Proline
Leucine
Isoleucine
Valine
Cofactors:
Vitamin B_1
Vitamin B_2
Vitamin B_6
Vitamin B_{12}
Vitamin C
Vitamin E
Folic acid
Vitamin B_3
Zinc

SEX AND STRESS

Besides the absence of specific sexual problems, sexual ability also depends upon the body's general state of well-being. Here, too, amino acids play a prominent role—particularly thanks to the aminos phenylalanine and tyrosine. Tyrosine combines with the mineral iodine in the thyroid gland to produce thyroxin, a hormone that controls your body's rate of cellular metabolism. Without sufficient thyroxin, the body becomes lethargic and sluggish. There is also a loss of interest in physical activity—including sex. Making sure your thyroid gland has enough tyrosine to produce thyroxin is vital in ensuring good health and, specifically, sexual activity. Phenylalanine also supports sexual activity through the metabolic pathway that affects the production of adrenalin.

Sexual performance is maintained by a complex interaction of two branches of the autonomic nervous system. While one branch, the sympathetic, is responsible for the fight-or-flight stress response, the other, the parasympathetic, is responsible for the body-at-rest functions, such as digestion. The two actually relate synergistically: It is the balance between the two systems that ensures adequate responses in a given situation. For example, even though the sympathetic nervous system prepares your body for the stress situation of sex by secreting adrenalin (which raises blood pressure and increases circulation to the lungs and muscles), if the stress becomes too great (perhaps because of extreme nervousness), the body will simply be unable to perform. Such are the complexities of balancing the para-sympathetic with the sympathetic branch of the autonomic nervous system. To maintain this balance and to respond evenly to the stress demands that sex makes on the body, a healthy circulating level of adrenalin is vital. For the stress response formula see page 102.

CARNITINE—THE DON JUAN AMINO

Another amino acid whose presence affects sexual performance is carnitine. Carnitine is needed to transport fatty acids into and out of the cellular membranes. It therefore plays a key role in ensuring that heart muscles are supplied with the energy that they need to respond even to the most extreme demands of lovemaking. Between 1 and 1.5 grams a day of L-carnitine should cover the benefits to be derived from this amino acid.

GENERAL FORMULA FOR SEXUAL HEALTH

We've looked at the uses of individual amino acids and formulas for specific sexual problems. Now let's look at a formula to improve general sexual health. This formula consists of combinations of free-form aminos with their vitamin and mineral cofactors. The nutrients should be taken in split doses throughout the day.

Aminos:
Histidine
Arginine
Lysine
Methionine

Phenylalanine
Tyrosine
L-carnitine
Cofactors:
Vitamin B_1
Vitamin B_2
Vitamin B_3
Vitamin B_6
Vitamin C
Pantothenic acid
Folic acid
Copper
Magnesium
Selenium
Zinc
Manganese
Iodine

Note: *Before taking any aminos, see Chapter 5, "Safety and Precautions."*

Overall high-level health is of immense importance in making sex work for you. Amino acids are basic to good health, contributing to all systems. In truth, our bodies are so finely balanced that the metabolic equilibrium is easily disrupted. When this happens, the body's functions begin to break down. Sexual disability is often a result of this fine metabolic disruption. To those who feel they are living in a prison of anxiety, bitterness, and bewilderment over sex, the right amino acids can be the key to freedom.

20

Help Against Herpes

"What's the difference between love and herpes?" "Simple. Herpes lasts forever." This joke is as old as the current herpes epidemic. It neatly sums up the reason for the sudden despair and isolation felt by many victims when they contract the virus. During an attack, this highly infectious, often excruciatingly painful virus brands victims with the physical stigma of lesions and cold sores, rendering the reassuring intimacy with a lover almost impossible without the threat of passing the infection on, regardless of precautions. And there is no known cure.

With their ability to strengthen the body's natural defenses, however, amino acids represent perhaps the most potent form of herpes prevention known. Even for those unlucky enough to have contracted the virus already, amino acid formulas are providing relief to thousands of victims. Let's see how herpes attacks the body. Then, by pinpointing the areas that it affects, we can formulate a metabolic program that will help to ease a sufferer's sense of isolation and agony.

Herpes infection takes two forms: simplex-one, which

affects the mouth with large, scabrous sores and blisters, and simplex-two, which affects the genitals in much the same way but often with intense pain. The herpes virus lives in the nerve cells. By attaching itself to the cell wall, it injects the cell with its own DNA. As DNA determines the characteristics of living things, this has the effect of adapting the nerve cell to obey the commands of the virus, allowing it to multiply. It spreads down the nerves to the skin, causing the highly infectious lesions to erupt on the surface. Each outbreak may last anywhere from a week to several months. Even when the lesions disappear and physical contact with a partner can be resumed without fear of passing on the infection, the virus is still present in the nervous system. It lies dormant, waiting until the metabolic conditions are ripe for it to spread again. Knowing what these metabolic conditions are, and why they allow the virus to prosper, is crucial in helping to decide which supplements to use.

STRESS AND HERPES

Doctors are finding that people most often contract herpes, and that symptoms recur in existing victims, following periods of stress. This is because the metabolic imbalances that stress causes deplete their bodies of the nutrients that provide them with natural immunity. Without a vigorous immune system to repel it, the virus can develop much more freely. Furthermore, finding you have contracted herpes is a highly stressful discovery in itself. The anxiety it causes can only lead to greater nutritional deficiencies. "I couldn't believe I'd caught it," said one victim. "I couldn't eat. I couldn't sleep. I was so worried. I thought, 'This is it. This is the end.' I was absolutely panic-stricken."

This attitude almost guarantees regular recurrences of the virus, for the last thing you can afford to do when you contract herpes is to squander your body's valuable metabolic resources by giving in to stress and anxiety. Uncontrolled stress is like a runaway train, relentlessly gathering speed and momentum. When the train finally hits the buffers at the end of the line, the impact is enormous. The same thing happens to a stressed body when it runs into an infection.

What you must try to do, instead of simply worrying, is to make sure that your body is equipped nutritionally to withstand the stress. We can protect our bodies from the physical and mental ravages of stress with amino acid supplements. This will leave us much more resistant to attacks from the herpes virus. So which nutrients provide the best protection? Glutamine will leave you much more alert and composed. As a brain fuel, it will help to alleviate the torpor and apathy of depression. This is crucial when you need all your energy and determination to fight the infection.

DL-phenylalanine, the precursor of tyrosine, is an antidepressant that almost literally charges your brain and body with adrenalin, the driving force of the stress response. DL-phenylalanine is also a proven painkiller and can give substantial relief against the pain of the herpes lesions. As pain itself is a major stressor, you can see that the help DLPA gives is vital.

Methionine is included in the formula because it is necessary for the conversion of noradrenalin to adrenalin. This formula may prove useful when taken three times a day between meals:

Aminos:
Glutamine
Tyrosine
DL-phenylalanine
Methionine
Cofactors:
Vitamin B_3
Vitamin B_6
Vitamin C
Magnesium

Note: *See Chapter 5, "Safety and Precautions," for the conditions under which to avoid phenylalanine and tyrosine.*

Mental Resistance

The preceding amino-based stress formula is one of the best nutritional support programs you can give your body. But it will be even more effective in strengthening your resistance to infection if you can raise your stress threshold. Experts now realize the importance of conditioning yourself not to feel stress in what might normally be a stress-causing situation. If, for example, you can sit in a traffic jam for hours, or be awakened at three in the morning by your neighbor's party without feeling anxiety or anger, then fewer essential nutrients will need to be diverted away from your immune system.

There are several methods of raising your stress threshold, which nutritionists are successfully using in conjunction with amino acid therapy. One very popular method is biofeedback. This is simply a method of learning to control the bodily processes that occur involuntarily, using the feedback of sensitive measuring instruments to guide you. For example, let's say you want to ease a migraine caused by stress. You might decide to attach to your hand a sensor that measures skin temperature. You would then try to imagine that the sun is shining on it—concentrating acutely on the feel of its imaginary warmth covering your skin. When the sensation becomes vivid, the capillaries in your hand will dilate. This happens because your body has been fooled into thinking that one small area is hotter than the rest. As your body wants to maintain an even temperature, it will pump blood to the skin surface to release heat. This in turn will lower the blood pressure in other parts of your body, including your forehead, and so relieve the migraine.

The biofeedback instrument itself provides no relief but, by showing the rise in skin temperature, acts as a guide in helping you develop your imaginative skill. With practice, you will find that you won't even need the equipment, and can ease your stress symptoms almost at will.

Another simple and effective method of stress control is meditation. According to the Friends of the Healing Research Trust, "meditation frees the mind from its enslavement to discursive thoughts with their attendant feelings which together dissipate energy and cause stress and suffering." Put aside 15 or 20 minutes a day to practice it at home. Sit quietly in a chair with your feet on the floor. Close your eyes, breathe deeply, and relax. Choose a simple word like *one*. Then, blocking out everything else—all your anxieties—repeat the word continuously to yourself. If you become distracted or feel your mind wandering, gently guide it back to the word and carry on repeating it.

Concentrating wholly on this word will seem impossible at first. Your mind will disobediently race from one preoccupation to another. If this happens, don't give up. Many patients who find they are easily distracted are encouraged to use the amino anxiety formula—tryptophan, histidine, glycine, and taurine—to help them. (See the complete high-anxiety amino formula on pages 108-9.)

The mind-relaxing effects of meditation or biofeedback coupled with the remarkable synergistic powers of the high-anxiety amino formula will help to heighten your resistance to infection. In turn, this reduces your chances of catching herpes.

If you have already been infected by the virus, controlling your stress in this way will help to inhibit the possibilities of further outbreaks. But raising your stress threshold in this way is a long-term prevention program.

THE HERPES WONDER-WORKER: LYSINE

There is one herpes treatment that is being used dramatically and effectively against the virus: the essential amino acid lysine. The possibility of using lysine to combat herpes has been explored since the early fifties. One particularly important piece of research was conducted by Dr. R. Tankersley. Working with a herpes virus growing in a culture dish, he found that the addition of arginine—an essential amino for the production of growth hormone—stimulated the virus. However, when he added the structurally similar amino lysine, the virus's growth was severely inhibited. Following this discovery, high doses of lysine were given to 45 herpes victims. Of these, 43 showed an astonishing improvement. The vesicles on their skin faded much more rapidly than normal, and the pain was much less. While they continued to take the lysine, no new lesions and blisters appeared. Lysine's effectiveness in treating the symptoms of herpes is now widely acknowledged. In the United Kingdom, for example, it is recommended by the Herpes Organization.

Arginine, on the other hand, actively encourages the growth of the virus (see Chapter 5). Therefore, to suppress the virus in your body, the ratio of arginine to lysine must be high in lysine's favor. During the active outbreaks of herpes lesions, you might take free-form lysine three times a day. This will help ease the pain and speed up the disappearance of the sores. You must be careful, though, not to deplete the arginine levels; inducing arginine deficiency by taking too much of the competing lysine may actually harm your immune response. Once the initial herpes outbreak diminishes, try to reduce your lysine dosage to keep the dormant virus in check. Better still, lysine can be bought as a cream. Simply apply it on the affected areas.

As well as the free-form powder of the cream, try to eat foods with a high lysine-to-arginine ratio. These include fish, chicken, beef, and lamb; milk, cheese, sprouts, beans, and most fruits and vegetables. At the same time, do your best to avoid the high-arginine foods: gelatin, chocolate, carob, coconut, whole wheat and white flour, nuts, and cereals.

HELP DURING BREAKOUTS

We scarcely give the metabolic cycle of our body a second thought. But in this, too, we have a powerful weapon in the fight against herpes. The body's metabolic cycle is composed of two opposing phases: anabolic and catabolic.

Once we know how these processes affect us, we can manipulate them into literally tearing the herpes infection down.

The anabolic and catabolic processes, you may remember, make up the continuous bodily cycle of life, death, and rebirth. When we are in an anabolic state, our bodies are growing and regenerating. Tissue repair, wound healing, and muscle buildup all happen anabolically. But at the same time, aspects of this part of the life cycle can also be harmful to the body. The growth of cancer tumors, the buildup of plaque in the blood, and the formation of moles and warts are also anabolic in nature.

The same thing is true of herpes, because the attack that the herpes virus mounts on the body—both in the nerve cells and on the skin surface—is a building-up process. It is anabolic. Therefore, if we can find a way of tilting the biochemical balance in favor of the body's catabolic— tearing down—phase, we can actually counter the anabolic attack of the virus.

Because they promote growth and regeneration, most amino acids are anabolic. Some, however, do behave catabolically, and we can use them to treat the herpes virus. They are methionine, cysteine, taurine, aspartic acid, and glutamic acid. Taken in a blend, they can actively inhibit the growth of the infection. Assisting the body's own catabolically based defenses, they will help it to tear down the viral inflammation when it occurs. A catabolic formula might look like this:

Aminos:
Methionine
Cysteine
Taurine
Aspartic acid
Glutamic acid
Cofactors:
Vitamin A
Vitamin B_6
Vitamin B_{12}

Vitamin C as calcium ascorbate
Folic acid
Magnesium aspartate

For maximum benefit, try to take this formula in the early
evening at the start of your catabolic cycle.

We've listed several methods for controlling the effects of
herpes. But do they work? For the answer, let's look at the
case of William, a teacher who came to us not long ago in
desperation. He had suffered a rash of painful sores some
years before which had been diagnosed by his doctor as
fungal growth. As the rash disappeared following a short
course of antibiotics, he had no reason to question the
doctor's diagnosis. Recently he became engaged. Amid the
chaos and stress of moving to a larger house and making
marriage arrangements, the rash reappeared. His fiancée
immediately contracted it, suffering unbearable vaginal
pain as a result. It was so debilitating, in fact, that she was
forced to take time off work. "I realized straight away it was
herpes," said William. "We both had it really badly. It was
as if our skin had been scraped raw and set on fire. Everyone
I spoke to said there was nothing we could do, that we just
had to live with it." Determined not to accept this, he came
for nutritional counseling.

Urinary amino tests showed that they were both suffering
from dangerously low amino acid levels almost across the
board. "There was so much to think about with the
wedding and everything. We were both eating out of cans
and were under a hell of a lot of stress." Accordingly, both
he and his fiancée were put on the full stress-control
program and prescribed high doses of supplemental lysine.
While the agonizing lesions persisted, they also took the
catabolic amino formula to help break down the sores.

The symptoms faded for both of them within 48 hours. "I
can't begin to describe the immense relief we felt," William
said later. "It made life seem twice as great." What it has
also done is to show William and his fiancée how important a healthy, nutritionally balanced lifestyle is, regardless

of whether they are threatened by illness. Because if you want to contain your herpes, you need a healthy body. Your digestion must be in good shape, you must be mentally stable, and you must be able to withstand stress without your metabolic pathways becoming depleted of nutrients. Natural vitality is the best weapon for fighting the virus. Without doubt, the free metabolic energy of amino acids represents the best way of achieving that vitality.

GENERAL WELL-BEING

Amino acids are the shock troops in the fight against herpes, but even they need logistical support. Make sure your intestinal tract has enough of the lactobacilli acidophilus and biffidus—the bacteria that are important for healthy digestion. They help break down the nutrients that the body needs for its stress response. They prevent allergic reactions from occurring in the intestines, as well as fighting the bowel-related mood disorders. You can find these bacilli in foods like yogurt and buttermilk or as tablet supplements. Zinc is also important for digestion. You need it for the formation of over 80 enzymes, and many of these are digestive enzymes. Zinc also helps you to fully absorb your food.

Eat as much fresh food as you can, especially fruit and vegetables. Try to get most of your fiber from these sources rather than from bran, which can easily irritate the intestines. Cut out as much carbohydrate as possible, and don't eat any refined food.

Finally, make sure you get sufficient vitamin C. This has so many roles in the body, from helping to build collagen to the infection-fighting protein interferon. The body needs it everywhere, and any small imbalance quickly creates stresses, particularly in your immune response.

Above all, don't be a helpless sufferer. The shock and stigma that people feel when they find they have herpes is enormous. It makes some withdraw from the human contact they need. Others try to boast about it as if they were wearing the latest Paris fashions. Neither of these attitudes is helpful. It's not a fashion or a cross to be borne but something you have to fight, actively and positively. If your life is stressful, if you eat poorly and rarely exercise, you are much more likely to contract it—or to endure greater suffering if you have it already. If, on the other hand, your lifestyle is healthy and balanced, then you already possess the best defense against herpes that we know of.

21

Free Aminos and Feeling Young

Hidden in the shadows of a dank, unlit attic sits a portrait in oils. Moving downstairs we spy the subject of this painting—a young, handsome man, perhaps in his late twenties. Engrossed in conversation with a friend, he speaks with the passion and vigor of his years. Yet, although the face of the young man and the face in the portrait belong to one and the same person, the figure in the portrait is old. Its cheeks are haggard and pale and creased; thin wisps of hair sit limply on the forehead, and folds of sallow skin sag from the throat. With each passing year this face grows a little more cadaverous, but the man downstairs—Dorian Gray—stays young, unbelievably young.

The notion of being able to stop the process of aging—and halt the inevitable decline toward death—occupies us all at some time. Of course, death is unavoidable, but there needn't be anything foregone about the way we age. Thanks to amino acids, we now have the power to slow down the aging process. Amino acid therapy refutes the traditional, deeply ingrained view that low energy and mental sluggishness, joint pains, loosening skin, and constant infection are the unavoidable results of aging. With the proper nutritional support, you can live a longer, fuller, and more vital life.

WHAT IS AGING?

One patient in his midfifties receiving nutritional counseling for arthritis described to us his feelings about aging: "To me, getting old is like finding yourself in a prison. You gradually realize that things you had taken for granted—like a good, strong body and the ability to think clearly—were actually only special privileges that have now been withdrawn."

To this man, getting older was an unbearably frustrating experience. It prevented him from being as active as he once was and caused the levels of adaptive energy in his body—the energy that allowed him to respond to stresses with vigor—to decline. Work became harder, and the mental effort to get things done greater. His concentration started to slip, and his memory to falter. Sexual activity declined. He suffered from periods of apathy, depression, and insomnia.

Perhaps the most common and harmful of all the consequences of growing old is that as a person ages, his digestive system gets lazy. Stomach acid production slows down dramatically even by the age of 40. And by 60 almost one person in three secretes no acid at all. When we lose stomach acid, the enzyme-making pancreas is forced to secrete additional enzymes to cope with these additional demands, yet the pancreas depends on stomach acid to stimulate the secretion of enzymes in the first place. The stress placed on the pancreas causes it to withdraw vitamins, minerals, and aminos from other functions, leaving the body vulnerable to a host of so-called age-related diseases such as arthritis, pneumonia, and reduced resistance to infection.

Because of this, many nutritionists believe that supporting the body's digestive system with nutritional supplementation is a vital part of helping you look and feel young.

THE DEMOLITION CREW

Another problem with aging is the action of free radicals. According to Pearson and Shaw in their book *Life Extension*, each quart of air contains a billion of these ravenous, destructive substances. Free radicals, as we have seen, are one of the main causes of allergies and many other illnesses, but when it comes to aging, they are particularly active. Let's see why.

In Chapter 1 we explained how fibrous protein chains weave together into the strong, flexible cables of collagen. We then saw how collagen molecules mesh with each other like the branches of a hedge, eventually forming tough, highly flexible organs such as the skin, heart, and blood vessels. If we were to look at these structures under a microscope, the dense interlocking network of collagen cables would resemble a massive builders' scaffolding. Now let's see what happens when a free radical forces its way into the structure. As long as the free radical has an unpaired electron, it possesses a positive charge, rather than the neutral charges of the molecules in the protein it has invaded. Therefore, to balance itself, the free radical attracts charges from surrounding molecules. But by robbing these charges from the collagen molecules, it breaks open the protein bonds and starts to dismantle the scaffolding-like molecules. This free-radical activity causes a chain reaction as molecules from the broken chains—now ravenous for electrons themselves—try to rob other, neighboring molecules of their electrons.

Now imagine just a fraction of the billion or more free radicals contained in one breath of air affecting your body. When two free radicals meet, a cross-linkage of destruction occurs, undoing whole sections of scaffolding. In time the collagen molecules will collapse like a demolished tower block.

Of course, this destruction takes place only on a microscopic level, and you won't suddenly find a pound of flesh falling off your arm (although free radicals are one of the causes of the dry flakiness of eczema). Instead, what you'll find is that your skin loses its softness and pliability and your face becomes gaunt, leathery, and wrinkled. A good test for free-radical activity is to pinch and lift the skin on the back of your hand, then let it go. If it springs back into place the skin is healthy, but if it is slow to return and retains a small, raised area where you pinched it, then nutritional support is almost certainly called for. Of course, it's not just your skin that depends on collagen. Free-radical activity damages capillaries as well, causing cardiovascular problems, restricting circulation, and preventing nourishment from reaching the cells. Similarly, it can attack the alveoli of the lungs, causing bronchitis and pneumonia. And it might alter DNA and RNA, leading to growths such as goiter and cancer.

Although free-radical activity itself is one of the major causes of aging, other factors allow the free radicals to take hold. The decline of digestive functions, with the resulting loss of enzyme production, is a major cause. The body manufactures two particular enzymes to keep free radicals in check: superoxidase dismutase (SOD) and glutathione peroxidase (GTP). Children who suffer from a genetic inability to manufacture these two particular enzymes are victims of the illness progeria, where the unfettered free radicals cause them literally to grow old and die, often before reaching adolescence. Supporting the pancreas with the materials it needs to create these antiaging enzymes has been shown to help victims of this awful disease. Many adults suffering from the same free-radical damage are finding similar relief by taking the complete amino blend.

THE WEIGHT DILEMMA

Another common cause of aging is a decline in the work rate of the endocrine organs. The most obvious symptoms of this are the loss of sexual appetite, decreasing growth hormone, fading levels of LH and FSH in women, and particularly a decline in the production of the immunity hormone thymosin. Perhaps even more important is the way that activity of the thyroid gland slows down. As you age and the production of thyroxin declines, the body needs fewer and fewer calories. Experts have estimated that after age 20 we need 1 percent fewer calories each year. A person celebrating his 70th birthday, therefore, needs only half the calories he would have needed 50 years earlier. On the other hand, his deteriorating physical state—poor digestion, reduced immunity—increases his body's need for the aminos, vitamins, and minerals found in his food.

This dangerous nutritional dilemma faces all of us as we grow older. We can continue eating the same amount of calories to obtain the nutrition we need, but in doing so risk heart disease, atherosclerosis, arteriosclerosis, and obesity when our food is metabolized inadequately. Or we can cut calorie intake by eating less, but starve our metabolic pathways of the nutrients they need for making protein structures.

Before we go on to see exactly how aminos can help, let's briefly sum up what we've covered so far: Aging is a process of degeneration caused by a complex corelationship of factors. The slowing of stomach acid production depletes the body's enzyme and immune systems. This leaves the body open to attack from infection and free-radical damage, which hastens the aging process. Much of the food eaten is used simply to support the beleaguered defenses, while tissue repair, sexual response, and general vitality all decline. At the same time, the slowing of hormone production prevents what food remains from being metabolized effectively, leading to weight increase as well as further starving the body of essential nutrients.

These are some of the problems facing people as they age. Looking at the way each symptom of aging contributes to the others, it's hard to tell where and how the process really starts. Does acid and enzyme depletion lead to an increase in free-radical activity, or vice versa? No one is quite sure. What is certain is that aging is a slow process, where recognizable symptoms gradually accumulate, and not some uncontrollable overnight metamorphosis. Hormone production declines gently; so do acid and enzyme secretion. Therefore, if you anticipate and attack the deficiencies almost before they occur with properly chosen amino acids and associated nutrients, you can stave off these symptoms. The skin's firmness can be prolonged and muscle tor.e retained; you can stay alert and active and free from disease much longer than you might ever have thought possible.

THE STAY-YOUNG AMINOS

So what sort of program should you follow? Remember that one of the most dangerous aspects of aging is the decline in digestive functions. The enormous strain this places on the enzyme and immune systems lowers resistance to disease and to the aging effects of free radicals. We saw in Chapter 17, "Digestive Troubles—A Thing of the Past," that one of the best ways to raise the levels of hydrochloric acid was with a dietary supplement of histidine, together with glutamic acid HCL, betaine HCL, and glycine. We've also seen the importance of a complete blend of amino acids in helping to relieve the stresses on the pancreas. It provides this most overworked of organs with additional amounts of all the raw materials it needs to fashion the protein-digesting enzymes.

Although they are the very building blocks of your body, free-form amino acids are also very low in calories. Therefore, while the complete blend will help to replace the protein lost as you age, it will do so without causing an increase in weight. This helps to get around that awkward nutritional dilemma caused by thyroxin depletion. With our normal diets, which are relatively high in carbohydrates and cholesterol, we pay for the protein by taking in fats and sugars at the same time. And while the endocrine system (particularly the thyroid gland) can metabolize this to release energy and promote muscle growth when we are younger, as we age these foods start to accumulate as fats. Taking much of the protein you need as free-form amino acids provides the necessary materials for maintaining muscle mass, replenishing worn-out protein in the organs, and providing new enzymes and hormones, without the fear of putting on weight.

ANTIAGING CHELATORS

Besides the complete blend and the acid-generating aminos, which other aminos should you take as part of a specific antiaging program? Heavy-metal toxicity poses such a threat to the body as it gets older that the chelating abilities of individual free-form aminos make powerful antiaging tools. The tripeptide amino glutathione (the combination of glycine, cysteine, and glutamic acid) is looked upon by nutritionists as a chelator *par excellence*. Experts find that it is effective in most cases of heavy-metal poisoning, and some factories in the United States are giving it to their workers to protect them against high emissions of lead and mercury in the air. These metals are notorious for causing irritability and short tempers, and some tests show that they suppress the immune system by oxidizing vitamin C. Glutathione works by transporting these harmful elements safely out of the body. Experts are currently using it to relieve nausea, hyperactivity, and emphysema. Its chelating ability is also being used with great success by arthritis sufferers.

Glutathione combines with the trace metal selenium to form one of the two natural free-radical scavenging enzymes, glutathione peroxidase (GTP). We've seen how important this and superoxidase dismutase (SOD) are in stifling the chain reaction of aging caused by free radicals. The immune system comes under severe testing in later life, and the support provided to it by glutathione makes it one of the most important aminos you can take.

Histidine not only supports stomach acid secretion and mediates your allergy response, it also is another excellent chelator. Besides glutathione and histidine, several other aminos also have a proven ability as chelators. They include methionine, cysteine, and aspartic acid. Whether you choose to include them in a specific formula or prefer instead to take them as part of the complete blend is up to you.

ENERGIZING YOUR BODY'S ANTIAGING PATHWAYS

While the chelator aminos work as a shield against the ravages of poisoning and free-radical damage, there are others you can take that will help to strengthen your body, raising it to an almost youthful level of efficiency. These are the aminos that supply and strengthen the endocrine organs and regenerate fading hormone levels. We saw in Chapter 9 how each of these aminos works. Ornithine stimulates the pituitary gland into releasing growth hormone (GH), which increases muscle synthesis and mobilizes fat deposits. At the same time, the amino tyrosine, together with cofactor iodine, raises the levels of thyroxin. When we are young, we can eat platefuls of food, because it is immediately burnt as energy or metabolized into muscle. This can happen because GH and thyroxin work synergistically to consume the food. Many people, anxious to recover lost muscle tone, have duplicated these youthful processes later in life by taking these two hormone-stimulating aminos. In addition, the amino carnitine, together with vitamin C, helps to mount a lipotrophic (fat-mobilizing) rearguard action, scouring for arterial fat buildup, and in doing so releasing more energy.

Another amino, arginine, is the precursor of spermine and spermidine. We've seen how these two chemicals relieve memory loss, surely one of the most disheartening aspects of aging. They also work as inhibitory nerve chemicals, suppressing the tremors and tics that are another sign of the aging process.

Another aging illness associated with motor dysfunction is Parkinson's disease. Although there is no cure, many victims are prescribed doses of the catecholamine neurotransmitter L-dopa; so you might include the precursor phenylalanine, together with tyrosine. We saw earlier how another problem of aging is a loss of adaptive energy (the inability to respond to stress), resulting in physical weakness as well as depression. In this case phenylalanine, as the precursor of noradrenalin and adrenalin, is a must. Another amino acid to include is tryptophan, beneficial for its calming effect. And cysteine is an amino that is becoming widely used to restore body to aging hair.

Of course, it's up to you which aminos you decide to include in an antiaging formula. Here, as a guide, are all the aminos we've mentioned in this chapter.

Aminos:
Histidine
Glutamic acid HCL
Glycine
Glutathione
Arginine
Ornithine
Phenylalanine
Tyrosine
Tryptophan
Methionine
Aspartic acid
Cysteine
Carnitine
Cofactors:
Vitamin A
Vitamin B_3
Vitamin B_6
Vitamin B_{12}
Folic acid
Vitamin C
Vitamin E
Betaine HCL
Zinc
Magnesium
Selenium
Calcium
Iodine

Don't forget that supplements of the complete blend, *as a foundation to whichever aminos you choose, will make an enormous difference.*

22

The Youthful Skin Connection

Skin is the single biggest organ of your body. Like any other organ, it plays a crucial role in the living process. It helps regulate body temperature and is an important part of the immune defenses, guarding against viral, fungal, and bacterial infection.

This chapter will focus on ways of using amino acids to keep your skin soft, moist, pliable, and looking young. Although the formulations we suggest are excellent for helping aging skin, they can be used to improve any skin problem: stretch marks, dry skin, or simply protection from ultraviolet light and pollution. Not just models and actors need good skin; we all do, and using free-form amino acids helps ensure that we have it.

AMINO SUNSPOTS

A hundred years ago, porcelain-white skin was thought to be one of the greatest assets of a beautiful woman. Today the darker the tan, the better. Although we find bronzed skin attractive, the damage that the sun's rays cause often far outweighs the benefits.

One of the most important factors in keeping your skin young-looking is the amount of moisture it retains. This is regulated by the prostaglandins, the chemicals derived from the unsaturated fatty acid linoleic acid. Prostaglandins have many roles in the body. They play a part in the immune response, and lubricate connective tissue. They also account for the natural oiliness of our skin. This oiliness works to retain billions of water molecules in the tissue, keeping it well irrigated.

When you lie on a blazing beach, no matter what factor of protective oil you apply, the sun's ultraviolet rays will penetrate the skin and start to oxidize these water molecules. This process robs water molecules of their electrons, and in doing so turns them into hydroxyls—the most dangerous of free radicals. When hydroxyl production reaches a certain level, it causes skin cancer. The destructive effect of ultraviolet light is a major reason for the scientific world's current concern over the loss of the ozone layer from the upper atmosphere. The ozone layer filters out most of the ultraviolet that comes from the sun, effectively protecting us from a hydroxyl-induced cancer epidemic. For without this layer—and there is already a hole in it the size of Antarctica caused by pollutants—the number of skin cancers would skyrocket.

You can use amino acids and their cofactors to provide you with effective hydroxyl protection. We saw in the last chapter how successful glutathione is as a free radical scavenger. Taken together with vitamins A and C, glutathione can protect the prostaglandins from free-radical damage. As heavy metals are another common cause of skin damage, the chelating ability of glutathione should make it a compulsory part of every Southern Californian's diet. Wherever you sunbathe, though, whether at Biarritz or Boston, it's well worth including glutathione in your diet. (As an alternative, you might prefer to use each of glutathione's less expensive constituent aminos: glutamic acid, cysteine, and glycine.) All are included in the healthy skin blend at the end of the chapter.

SULPHUR-BASED SKIN SUPPORT

Staying in California for a moment, there are days in Los Angeles when the smog becomes so dense that, with the sun shining bleakly through, it casts an orange-yellow glow on everything. This is due to the high levels of sulphur in the smog, which comes from the sulphur in car exhaust fumes. Sulphur is one of the natural by-products of burning fossil fuels. The effect that power station emissions—also high in sulphur—are having on the rivers, lakes, and forests of Scandinavia and Germany is currently the subject of a major political controversy in Europe. One recent scientific conference revealed that sulphuric acid raining on the Black Forest in Bavaria has already destroyed one tree in four. This is ironic: As far as your skin is concerned, the revitalizing powers of sulphur are second to none. It protects against radiation, oxidation, heavy metals, and hydroxyls, and has been recognized for centuries as one of the best substances you can take to revitalize tired skin.

Supplements of the sulphur-based aminos—methionine, cysteine, and taurine—will provide sulphur in concentrated and easily assimilated forms. Of these three aminos, experts find that cysteine is the most effective in relieving skin problems. This isn't surprising, as a quarter of all the amino acids contained in collagen (the skin protein) are cysteine molecules. Without them, collagen would simply fall apart. This is because cysteine's sulphur atoms link with each other in the spiral collagen helixes to form strong, flexible bonds, and these bonds help maintain the helix structure. If you were to compare a collagen helix with a spiral staircase (their shapes are very similar), then each step of that staircase would be a cysteine bond, keeping the spiral shape intact. The free-radical-generated oxidation process that causes the skin to age works by undoing these bonds, making the spiral fall apart.

By ensuring that the body has enough cysteine—in effect, by flooding your metabolism with it—you can actually quench the free-radical craving for the electrons in these bonds and prevent them from damaging the skin. Indeed, nutritionists often refer to cysteine and glutathione as "free-radical quenchers"—a phrase that actually sums up their role more accurately than the commonly used "scavenger." (See page 196 for a healthy skin formula.)

FLEXIBLE SKIN

Stretch marks are usually associated with pregnancy, but in fact they affect many people besides expectant mothers. These scarlike ribbons of diaphanous skin are responsible for a great deal of self-consciousness and anxiety.

Gary, a musician in his early twenties, complained of stretch marks that he had acquired as a result of weight lifting. "Every time I did a really good, hard workout I could feel my skin literally tearing," he said. Rolling up his sleeves, he uncovered his upper arms revealing what looked like tiny, broken strands of silver on his skin.

Stretch marks occur when the skin hasn't the elasticity to expand. Although it might feel perfectly pliable to the touch, the rigidity occurs at the molecular level. It often signifies a dietary deficiency of many important nutrients, particularly tryptophan and zinc. Zinc is the most important trace element in collagen. It lends the skin pliability and strength, and to protect against further stretch marks, many nutritionists recommend taking it as a supplement along with tryptophan. Why take these two together? Basically, tryptophan helps ensure that zinc is carried through the intestinal wall into the bloodstream.

As well as tryptophan, we also recommend glycine as part of a blend to prevent stretch marks. There are, in fact, even more molecules of glycine in each collagen chain than there are of cysteine. Glycine is a tiny amino acid that works in the collagen chains like the springs in a car, absorbing the stresses and allowing it to flex without damage. Glycine deficiency makes the collagen very brittle: some experts believe that this lack of "give" is what leads to the sudden rupture of a stretch mark.

Within a few weeks of starting to take these supplements, together with the complete blend, Gary's skin had stopped tearing, and the existing marks were starting to clear up. (See below for a healthy skin formula.)

SKIN HEALING

Another form of skin damage that aminos help heal are the minor cuts and bruises of everyday life. Any wound, no matter how small, depletes the levels of arginine from the body's supplies. The lower the level sinks, the longer a wound will take to heal—especially if arginine is diverted into other functions such as supporting the immune system.

Judith, a graphic designer, told us what happened when she accidentally cut her hand with a paper cutter while trimming some card stock. As soon as it happened, she bathed the wound, bandaged it, and expected it to heal. Unfortunately, soon after this she caught a virus from her boyfriend. With most of the available nutrients in her body fighting the virus, there was little left of the amino pool to help the wound. As a result, starved of the nutrients it needed for repair, the cut became livid, swollen, and painful.

At first she took the antibiotics her doctor prescribed, but when these only gave her a headache, she came for nutritional counseling. Her hand by now had become so swollen that she was unable to bend her fingers. Her lymph nodes, too, were swollen, showing that her immune system was under great stress. She was immediately given the complete amino blend to stimulate the immune system. In addition, she was given extra supplements of arginine, glycine, and cysteine to help the wound heal. Within a few days, the swelling had disappeared, and by the end of the following week, the large red weal it left had also gone.

For ensuring good, healthy skin—whatever complaint you suffer from—try this combination twice a day:
Aminos:
Complete bend
Glutathione
Glutamic acid

Cysteine
Tryptophan
Glycine
Arginine
Cofactors:
Vitamin A
Vitamin B$_3$
Vitamin B$_6$
Vitamin C
Zinc

VITILIGO

Another skin problem that responds to dietary supplementation with the complete amino blend is vitiligo. This is a disease that mainly affects people of Afro-Caribbean and Indian origin, destroying the pigment in their skin. It leaves large and unsightly white areas and is a source of distress and anxiety. Experts think that, by raising enzyme production in the body, the complete blend will help stimulate those enzymes responsible for the metabolic pathways of pigmentation.

One of the molecules needed for the pigment melanin is phenylalanine, and nutritionists speculate that using it together with folic acid and the complete blend will halt the spread of vitiligo. It may even help replace the pigment that has been lost.

As you can see, amino acids help to relieve a variety of skin-related problems. Here are some additional suggestions:

▶ The complete blend, along with arginine and cysteine, helps reduce acne and boils.

▶ If you suffer from eczema, the allergy combination of histidine and glutathione will help to clear it.

▶ Cold sores respond excellently to lysine—you can buy it as a cream and apply it directly to the affected area, as well as taking it orally in capsule or powder form.

Skin complaints are more public than most health problems. Short of hiding away, a victim of acne, eczema, or loss of pigmentation can't prevent the problem from being noticed. Happily, many people with skin complaints are unaffected by the anxiety that this problem causes others. Even so, in spite of this positive attitude, no one should ever feel they must settle for poorly conditioned skin.

We know well enough by now that any health problem you have is only a symptom of a much wider metabolic imbalance throughout your body.

In this respect, the approach you take for revitalizing damaged or aging skin is no different from the way you treat any other health disorder. Whether you use amino acids simply to protect your skin from ultraviolet light or as part of an antiwrinkling program, they will support your entire body by treating it for what it is: a single organism with thousands of interrelated pathways.

23

Amino First Aid

So far, we've seen how amino acids can help restore disrupted metabolic pathways that cause mental, emotional, and physical illness. Since this is a slow healing process, amino acids and their cofactors usually take some time to effect relief. It might take a few days, a few weeks, or—if the illness is a serious one such as heart disease—a few months before the full benefits are felt throughout the entire body. Because of the slow, cumulative effects of these supplements, you probably wouldn't expect them to be used for cases that demand immediate treatment. In fact, the opposite is true.

To show why, this chapter looks at the benefits of giving amino acids to victims of accidents or injuries. Prompt treatment—providing immediate emotional and physical support—is crucial in those first moments following a trauma such as a car accident, bereavement, mugging, or even rape. The sort of help the victim receives will play a major role in determining how quickly he or she recovers.

AMINO SHOCK TROOPS

Perhaps the most effective use of amino acids for first-aid care is the way they protect the body from shock. In fact, if your metabolic pathways are well supplied, your body can probably resist shock altogether. However, if you are unlucky enough to be a shock victim, there are blends you can take that will help offset its worst effects. Before we see what they are, let's first look at what is meant by shock.

Shock is a violent response to sudden stress—physical, mental, or emotional. We've all experienced the conditions that lead to this stress at some time in our lives. For example, when a dog runs out into the road and you have to slam on the brakes for an emergency stop, your heart palpitations and sudden perspiration are symptoms of mild shock. It's the same if you catch a flap of the stair carpet with your toe and fall downstairs. Even your startled reaction to a horror film is a form of shock. Each of these examples leaves you with a racing heartbeat, a queasy feeling in your stomach, and a sudden sense of weakness and shivering.

These unpleasant physical sensations are, of course, the results of your body's sympathetic—fight or flight—nervous system. The diversion of blood away from the stomach to the heavy muscles causes the nauseous sensation in your stomach, and the pounding heartbeat is the effort of your body to provide those muscles with the oxygen they need to perform. Meanwhile, the level of beta-wave activity in your brain rises dramatically. This increases your alertness, allowing you to decide on a quick and efficient reaction—you are literally prepared to fight or take flight from the circumstances that caused the stress. You are aware of everything around you, sensitive to the slightest change, and ready to respond. This response is so far outside the body's normal functions that it places quite a strain on its resources.

Usually the fight-or-flight reaction is short-lived and mild enough to leave you with nothing but a sense of fatigue. You might feel emotionally drained, but nothing worse.

Sometimes, though, people are plunged into situations where a much more extreme response is demanded, and this response may upset the sympathetic/parasympathetic balances altogether.

Kathy, herself a nutritionist, described an accident in which she was involved. She was a passenger in a car that hit a patch of black ice on the road, skidded, and rolled down an embankment. "Looking back on it, I realize how acutely aware I was of what was happening. I remember watching the grass and the horizon revolve in slow motion—not just as a blur; I swear I saw every blade of grass. I also remember noticing a cloud in the sky that resembled one in a print I have at home." Kathy's acute, dreamlike awareness—as if her senses had suddenly been amplified—is a typical effect of the sympathetic nervous system. The mind becomes highly alert and active. In fact, this alertness functioned far beyond her conscious state. "I wasn't aware of my body at all," she continued. "It's as if it took care of itself without any conscious help from me." When Kathy tried to recall how she had clawed her way out of the overturned car, her mind was a blank. This highlights another aspect of the shock-related stress response: Kathy's reasoning ability was subordinated to her instinct—the instinct for survival.

Luckily, being a nutritionist, Kathy had well supplied her body with all the nutrients necessary for supporting these stress demands, and she experienced no shock afterward. For many people caught in this sort of situation, though, the sudden, extreme physical reaction has more lasting effects. It prevents digestion and protein synthesis, slows down enzyme production, and impedes the immune system. It can also result in chronic mood disorders. This is exactly what happens to many victims of shock. The immediate results may be stupor, torpor, and unresponsiveness—or alternatively, extreme anxiety, perhaps even hysteria. Later it may lead to widespread nutritional deficiencies in the body, which in turn can lead to illness, infection, and degeneration. Shock kills.

As shock is only an extreme form of stress, one of the

most important aims of first aid must be to administer sound nutritional support, particularly in the form of amino acids. So which aminos should you use? As we've seen, the shock trauma is likely to cause imbalances and blockages throughout the metabolic pathway network. Doses of a complete amino blend should therefore be included as the first line of defense against its effects. The complete blend will protect against enzyme depletion and support the immune system.

Then, a blend that will calm the victim is important for helping to guard against long-term stress damage. The amino anxiety formula—tryptophan, histidine, glycine, and taurine—is ideal for calming the patient in this way (see pages 108-9 for the complete anxiety formula).

In the longer term, you'll want to guard against post-shock depression. Like any stress—good as well as bad—shock will leave you drained of the nutrients you need for an adequate response to further stresses. When we've been under pleasant stress, the loss of the stressor—perhaps the excitement of a special vacation—leads to a sense of anticlimax and melancholy. The same is true for the aftereffects of shock. After expending so much energy and so many essential nutrients in responding to the situation (first by engaging the sympathetic nervous system and then by enduring the prolonged stress-related depletion of shock), your body is left with little for the necessary responses to the simple, everyday activities such as working, socializing, and even getting up in the morning. You might sink into depression. Every action will become an effort, and concentration will seem impossible. This might also be compounded by an anxiety neurosis, an abiding fear of whatever it was that caused the shock. So providing your body with the nutrients that help it to rise to the normal demands of life is important.

The most effective of these nutrients are the aminos phenylalanine and tyrosine and the brain fuel glutamine. As basic shock support, though, we recommend the following nutrients, taken twice a day until you feel they are no longer needed.

Aminos:
Complete blend
Tryptophan
Histidine
Glycine
Taurine
Phenylalanine
Tyrosine
Glutamine
Methionine
Cofactors:
Vitamin B_3
Vitamin B_6
Vitamin C

PHYSICAL INJURY

As well as providing emotional and mental support, amino supplements can also be used to help the victims of physical injury. The trauma of injury and the demands it makes on the body's supply of aminos, vitamins, and minerals leads to nutritional depletion as rapidly as psychological stress. Arginine is one of the first aminos that should be given to an injured patient. Arginine also supports the thymus gland. The thymus-generated immune response is crucial in preventing infection from entering through the injured skin. The sulphur-based aminos (particularly cysteine), together with taurine, will also aid skin repair.

If muscle damage has occurred, then it's best to add supplements of the branched-chain amino acids—leucine, isoleucine, and valine—to the formula. Any muscle injury depletes the available supplies of the branched-chain amino group.

Some nutritionists also give the branched-chain aminos,

together with arginine (in its role as the stimulator of growth hormone) and tyrosine (the precursor of thyroxin) to the victims of broken limbs. When a limb is set, it is encased in plaster, perhaps for many months. Unfortunately, the muscle that surrounds it tends to atrophy through disuse. Because of this, even after the plaster is removed, the patient must often undergo a further tedious period of rehabilitation, exercising the limb to promote a full return of muscle tone. But now, thanks to amino supplementation, experts feel that this muscle atrophy may be slowed or even prevented.

For physical trauma, try these supplements twice a day:

Aminos:
Complete blend
Arginine
Methionine
Cysteine
Taurine
Tyrosine
Leucine
Isoleucine
Valine
Cofactors:
Vitamin A
Vitamin B_3
Vitamin B_6
Vitamin B_{12}
Vitamin C
Zinc
Calcium

For the bone itself, the best supplement to take is a complete amino blend. Bone is made with a latticework of protein scaffolding, into which is mounted calcium phosphate. The proteins depend on a host of enzymes and aminos for their manufacture, and any depletion can easily slow down the healing process. If, for example, the patient hasn't received full nutritional support to guard against the shock of the injury, then the bone may mend a lot more slowly than the bone of a patient who has this support.

PROTECTION FROM INFECTION

Most of the book has concerned itself with ways of using free-form aminos to help relieve a variety of preexisting health problems. However, using these marvelous supplements only *after* you have a problem greatly underestimates their potential. By strengthening the body's immune defenses, amino acids can be used to stop many illnesses—particularly infections—from occurring in the first place.

When a virus first invades your body, long before symptoms of the infection actually appear, the immune system, led by its T-cell lymphocytes, swings into action. When the invading virus is relatively insignificant, the immune system is able to deal with it easily by using readily available supplies of amino acids and cofactors. The chances are that you won't even be aware of this minor infection.

Every now and then you come into contact with stronger, more virulent strains of viruses. This puts far greater demands upon the immune system. Accordingly, the response must be much stronger. But often there simply isn't a deep enough pool of circulating aminos to provide this massive response immediately. It takes time for the body to marshal its resources. While the body is assembling its forces, the virus is free to take hold. Consequently, you come down with an illness and have to endure a slow recovery period, as the immune system only gradually comes to grips with the infection.

However, if you can raise the circulating levels of the amino acids needed for the immune response when you first come into contact with the infectant, you will stand a far better chance of resisting illness. Free-form amino acids encourage the immune system to provide an immediate response. Of course, often you don't realize that you've been infected until you actually start showing symptoms. But there are other occasions—during a flu epidemic, for example—when, by taking the complete blend, you can strengthen your immune system to a point where it might successfully repel the virus. Many people take the complete blend and cofactors every day for just this sort of protection. Of course, if you *do* come down with an infection, the complete blend will also help speed your recovery, especially if you recognize the symptoms in their early stages.

TOXICITY TAMERS

The phrase *environmental toxicity* covers a lot of ground, but perhaps the most topical concern is radiation poisoning. The recent fears caused by Chernobyl and persisting doubts about the safety of nuclear plants in the West have led more and more people to nutritional supplementation to protect themselves from radiation. For example, news reports told how quickly chemists' stocks of iodine disappeared after the Chernobyl reactor explosion. As one of the main components of thyroxin, it helps to guard against thyroid cancer (caused by irradiated iodine) by saturating the thyroid with unradiated iodine. In fact, there are many other supplements that we can take for protection. The following amino free-radical scavengers are particularly effective:

Aminos:
Glutathione
Methionine
Cofactors:
Vitamin B_3
Vitamin B_6
Vitamin C
Zinc
Magnesium
Iodine

In addition to radiation, the levels of conventional pollution seem to grow each year. The heavy metals that billow into the atmosphere from factory chimneys and car exhausts prevent your body from absorbing many of the vital trace elements. We've seen how chelation therapy combats this, using aminos to get rid of damaging heavy metals by clamping onto them and making it easy for the body to remove them. These chelator aminos—methionine, cysteine, and glutathione—also make excellent supplements if you are caught near a factory fire, or if you have to work in an environment high in heavy-metal toxicity.

As we've seen, it's almost impossible to impose boundaries on the health-enhancing potential of amino acids. Admittedly, when you give first aid to a victim, it's tempting to concentrate on the symptoms or the immediate effects of shock or injury and ignore the longer-term consequences. Often, though, the seeds of further illness and degeneration are sown because of this attitude—that is, of course, unless full nutritional supplementation is provided as a component of the overall first-aid program. With these nutrients, you can ward off the emotional and psychological disorders of shock, support the body against any deficiencies that may result, and help to speed up wound healing.

PART SIX
CONFRONTATION WITH COMPULSION

24

Put Out the Smoke with Amino Acids

The scene is a crowded North African nightclub. A pianist sings a plaintive lament to lost love. At his side sits a beautiful woman who gazes wistfully into space. The owner of the nightclub enters and, seeing the woman, his eyes narrow in a mixture of pain and wryness. Half mumbling, he utters one of the most famous lines of the century: "Of all the gin joints in all the towns in all the world, she has to come into mine."

Casablanca is one of the world's great films. It is also arguably one of the most subversive. Next time you watch it, see how the everpresent use of cigarettes is employed as a vital dramatic component. There is a great emotive charge in watching Bogart nonchalantly light up (his face chiseled in highlight and shadow by the match flame), caught as he is between his love for Bergman and the danger of the Nazis. The rest of his world may be coming apart, but at least he can fall back for stability on his Gauloises. His smoking seems to make his situation at once more realistic and more romantic. Yet today, smoking is one of the world's biggest killers. Anyone who thinks it enhances their image or, worse, that it gives them physical or emotional support, is living in a *Casablanca* dream world.

Amino acids can't miraculously make you stop smoking—you must really want to do that yourself. But if you do stop smoking, you will find amino acids an invaluable aid in helping to ease the cravings that will follow. And more, they will give your body back the nutritional support it needs to recover from the damage that smoking causes— improving your digestion, circulation, and concentration, and generally revitalizing your life.

THE KILLER ALIGHT

If you smoke, you are one of nearly eighty million smokers in the United States alone. Of this number, 80 percent of men and 60 percent of women consume at least one pack a day, despite the overwhelming evidence that shows it causes lung, stomach, and bladder cancer; bronchitis; influenza; ulcers; and heart disease. If you smoke heavily, there is a good chance that large fat deposits are forming in your blood now, hardening your arteries and raising your blood pressure. Normally our bodies stop this from happening. Zinc, for example, is used by the body to keep arteries in good condition. But cadmium, a heavy metal found in cigarette smoke, displaces zinc. The lungs also need zinc to maintain their elasticity, which is why so many smokers— their lung tissue starved of zinc—suffer from emphysema.

Smoking causes an excess in your blood of another natural opponent of zinc: copper. A small amount of copper is needed for hemoglobin, the oxygen-carrying blood cells. But larger amounts destroy vitamin C. Vitamin C deficiency (and 25 mg of vitamin C are destroyed with each cigarette) raises blood pressure, leading to heart attacks and strokes and making your skin age prematurely.

Excess copper also creates an enzyme that breaks down the highly active amino histamine. Without enough histamine, your body won't produce sufficient stomach acid to digest your food properly. Your immune system will succumb to infection more easily. As well as losing your sex drive, you might fall prey to anxiety or schizophrenia.

The carbon monoxide that is released when your cigarette burns destroys brain cells by starving them of oxygen. Nicotine also interferes with the release of hormones. By raising insulin secretion from the pancreas, it robs the brain of its major fuel, glucose (the other being the amino glutamine). This often causes fatigue and dizzy spells and may even result in low blood sugar. Nicotine also causes up to an 80 percent increase in blood adrenalin levels. At first this might make you anxious and nervous. Later, as the adrenalin levels begin to drop, it will exhaust you, and might even lead to chronic depression.

The degeneration that smoking causes accumulates slowly in the body, so slowly that you might not notice the loss of taste in your food, the poor digestion, your developing night blindness, your short temper, the anxiety, even the difficulty you have breathing. Not notice, that is, until you stop smoking and realize the difference.

If you smoke, you probably get tired of pious nonsmokers lecturing you about giving up. (You might have your own reasons for smoking which they refuse to understand.) Even if you do want to stop, these reasons will play heavily on your mind. So before we look at how to give it up, let's examine the arguments you might give for continuing to smoke.

WHY YOU SMOKE

One reason for smoking—particularly when you start and the novelty is fresh—is the thought that it enhances your appearance. Does it? Recently we watched a ten-year-old playing football in a playground. Every so often he took a drag from the cigarette he held between his thumb and forefinger, closing his eyes each time as if in rapture. He was acting the role of the nonchalant male and must have thought he looked marvelous. What he looked was absurd. No one needs to act a part at all—and to do it by polluting your body is tragic.

Smoking also allows you to waste time. You might take a drag on your cigarette before answering a question; it gives you time to gather your thoughts. Then there is the tactile quality of your cigarette. It is something to hold on to, to fidget with. "If I'm at a stand-up party," said one smoker, "I must have a drink in one hand and a cigarette in the other so I won't feel awkward."

People also imagine that cigarettes relieve tension. They're wrong. What relaxes you is the stretching of your lungs as you take a drag rather than the actual inhaling of the tobacco. Watch people when they are tense and frightened: They gasp or sigh involuntarily to relieve their anxiety. In other words, you will get as much relief just from breathing deeply.

Last is the addiction. Your body quickly gears itself to the abnormal demands that smoking makes (such as increasing the blood adrenalin levels). Stopping suddenly disorients the metabolism. You become nervous, drowsy, anxious; you suffer from loss of energy, sweating, cramps, tremors, and palpitations. Put simply, you need a nicotine fix. Paradoxically, this is one of the factors that makes smoking so attractive. Because, unlike most areas of our lives, it is a desire that you can easily meet. "Simply by lighting up, I'm achieving a little victory against adversity," said one smoker, "So why should I stop?"

These reasons, the last especially, are what makes smoking such a difficult habit to give up. However, if you really do want to stop, you can. Let's see how to cope with the physical and mental addiction. Then we'll examine the way amino acids, minerals, and vitamins can help you stop smoking.

STARTING TO STOP

Once you have decided that you want to give up cigarettes, don't get carried away. You must remember that when you first started you probably smoked only now and then, rather than the pack or more a day that you smoke now. Consequently, your physical and psychological dependence will have grown slowly, the destructive effects accumulating almost unnoticed. If you don't realize how nicotine-dominated your body is, you will probably try to give up smoking totally in one go. This is too drastic. It almost always leads to acute withdrawal symptoms as the body is suddenly deprived of nicotine. The anxiety and craving that result might well drive you straight back to the cellophane-wrapped pack.

Instead, what you should do is slowly and methodically cut out cigarettes from particular times of your day. Then, using the remarkable calming and strengthening powers of amino acids, prepare yourself to withstand the withdrawal symptoms when they happen. In this way you can control the cravings, rather than allowing them to control you.

First, think of all those activities that involve lighting a cigarette: speaking on the phone, driving to work, drinking a cup of coffee. Choose one, and then stop yourself from ever lighting up in that situation again. Gradually widen the list of smoking-excluded activities so that finally there are only small pockets left in your day when you can smoke. Then, when you do smoke, take no more than three drags from the cigarette. This will satisfy your addiction without actually strengthening it.

No matter how slow this process is, your body will start reacting to the physical changes. You might suffer from periods of fatigue or excess energy. Your head will start to ache, and you will feel sick. You will probably start fretting and feeling sorry for yourself. The pressure to smoke will be intense, not helped by friends at work, smoky bars, and devious advertising gimmicks. You will pass through phases of depression, resentment, and anger. This is where amino acids really come into their own: By promoting a more tranquil and relaxed state of mind, they will leave you better able to cope with the anguish of withdrawal.

Helpers

Histidine is probably the most beneficial amino you can take to help you overcome your cravings. Taken as a supplement, it helps to relieve your anxiety and fretfulness, leaving you more composed, relaxed, and objective.

As the precursor of serotonin, the amino acid tryptophan makes another excellent dietary supplement when you stop smoking. Research measuring the brain waves of volunteer patients shows that about 45 minutes after taking tryptophan and its conversion in the body to serotonin, their waking states become more relaxed and tranquil. This helps you through the parts of the day you stop smoking: you can take a tryptophan supplement in advance to ease the anxiety you feel when you stop. When you take tryptophan, you will probably find that it extends the periods you can go without cigarettes for much longer throughout the day. Unlike synthetic tranquilizers, it won't interfere with your work by making you drowsy.

Smokers often find they are helped by taking the entire anxiety formula, which you will find at the end of this section and which also includes histidine to help stop cravings. Roger, a former heavy smoker, is the owner of a small lumber yard. His stockyard is accessible only through a narrow alley, and as there is no room to turn in the yard, he has to reverse his truck up the alley when he delivers or collects materials. It's a skillful and physically demanding maneuver, with only inches to spare on either side. He has to be alert and sensitive to the handling of the truck. "It annoyed me," he said, "because once my truck was in the yard, the first thing I did was put a cigarette in my mouth. I realized that any pressure on me, like reversing in here, made me immediately light up. I'd been thinking of giving up for some time, so I finally decided to give it a go. The trouble was that when I did give it up, I got short-tempered really easily, and I became forgetful and clumsy. When it came to reversing up that alley, I was terrible. I just couldn't keep a straight line. I kept overcompensating with the steering wheel so that I scraped first one wall then the other. When I reached the yard, my hands were shaking and I was gasping for a cigarette." Luckily, instead of giving in to the anxiety, the mental instability, and the physical lack of coordination, he followed a friend's advice and tried the amino anxiety formula. It did the trick. He hasn't smoked since, and neither has his truck scraped the alley walls.

Here's the formula:

Aminos:
Tryptophan
Histidine
Glycine
Taurine

Cofactors:
Vitamin B_1
Vitamin B_2
Vitamin B_6
Vitamin C
Calcium
Zinc

Depression

In addition to the sort of anxiety felt by Roger, many smokers have to weather periods of torpor and depression when they give up smoking. It's as if, without cigarettes, they simply have no will or energy of their own. Remember that nicotine can cause massive increases in the circulating levels of adrenalin. This is the end product of the body's excitory stress pathway, and continual stimulation effectively turns you into an adrenalin junkie. So when the levels begin to sink, you will almost certainly feel depressed. Without the nicotine stimulant, you might find it hard to respond to stress when you have to. Smokers often say that cigarettes pick them up—the fact is that cigarettes create the depression in the first place.

The aminos phenylalanine and tyrosine are the best supplements to take when you feel like this. They help replenish circulating levels of noradrenalin and adrenalin. Methionine—taken with phenylalanine and tyrosine to help the conversion of noradrenalin to adrenalin—is also a highly effective aid in picking you up. (See the blend at the end of this chapter.)

Sugar Problems

Another cause of depression may be connected with your insulin levels. Insulin is the hormone produced in the pancreas that regulates the amount of sugar that the body and brain receive. Nicotine fools the body into thinking that there is more sugar circulating than there really is. Insulin is then secreted to lower these phantom blood sugar levels by encouraging the liver to store the sugar. In fact, since your sugar levels are probably normal, this storage process will dangerously reduce them. The result can be dizziness, faintness, irritability, nervousness and, of course, depression.

Recently a research team found that blood sugar levels can be regulated by certain free-form amino acids. They discovered that the aminos glutamine, glycine, and lysine raise blood sugar levels. These aminos are now widely used to relieve cases of low blood sugar, particularly from cases of postsmoking depression. Furthermore, glutamine is a brain fuel in its own right—it heightens your alertness and allows you to think more clearly. (See the blend at the end of this chapter.)

Getting Better

Unlike conventional drugs, amino acids work synergistically—when taken to strengthen one metabolic pathway, they help strengthen many others. So when you take these aminos, they won't just help you to fight the cravings, anxiety, tension, fatigue, and depression; they will also prove invaluable in helping your body recover from the biochemical damage of smoking. Your digestion will improve. Food will taste so good you might think that up until now you had been wearing a sock over your tongue. Your improving physical well-being (at a drastically faster rate thanks to amino acid supplements) will naturally add momentum to your desire to give up smoking totally.

CIGARETTES AND WEIGHT GAIN

For many ex-smokers, one of the most distressing results of stopping is finding that, without cigarettes, they tend to put on weight quickly. There are several reasons for this:

▶ For one, the stress that giving up smoking causes elicits a response from the sympathetic nervous system. One way to counter this is to eat more.

▶ Many people, without realizing it, eat when they are anxious— whether it is about failing their driving test or giving up smoking.

▶ Others use eating as a substitute for the time wasting that they used to get away with by smoking. When you stop, you suddenly find yourself with a lot of spare time, and it must be tempting to fill it by eating an extra snack or two.

▶ With your digestion improving as a result of giving up smoking, you will probably feel hungrier. You might have to eat more at mealtimes just to feel sated.

▶ Smoking creates abnormal fatty acids in your system. These fatty acids are catabolic (destructive). Your body responds by manufacturing anabolic steroid output to counteract them. When you stop smoking, you stop the influx of abnormal fatty acids, but your body is still manufacturing the anabolic steroids for awhile—often making it difficult for you to keep weight off.

These factors tend to act upon each other, making the weight gain sometimes dramatic. To prevent this from happening, many nutritionists have found phenylalanine to be a marvelous appetite suppressant. Taken at bedtime, phenylalanine can help to reduce your cravings for sweets and snacks between meals.

Carnitine is another amino that helps to prevent weight gain. It is used to stimulate fat metabolism in patients suffering from obesity.

When all is said and done, the hardest thing about giving up smoking is to convince yourself that you need to. Every fact, every awful detail about the havoc it wreaks in your body won't make the slightest difference unless you truly want to stop.

If you do make the decision to stop, you can depend on

amino acids to help you overcome the enormous hurdle of physical and mental cravings with this formula:

Aminos:
Phenylalanine
Tyrosine
Methionine
Glutamine
Glycine
Lysine
Carnitine
Cofactors:
Vitamin B_3
Vitamin B_6
Vitamin C
Vitamin D
Zinc

Note: *Before taking either of the formulas in this chapter, see Chapter 5, "Safety and Precautions."*

25

The Alcohol-Amino Link

"It's been awful. He was fired from his job about four months ago because of his drinking. He's in his late forties and his boss refuses to give him a reference, so even if he does come off the bottle he's virtually unemployable. We've had to sell the house, and we're up to our neck in debt. I'm working as a waitress in a coffee shop—it's the only income we've got coming in. He's no help at all. The other day he said, "I'm just popping out to buy a paper," as charmingly and breezily as possible. Three hours later, I got a call from a bar owner asking me to come and collect my husband. He was leaning against the bar dead drunk, and when he saw me come in, he said, "Oh, here she is. Madam high and mighty. Why don't you leave me alone?" This was in front of a bar full of regulars. He just doesn't realize how cruel he is. If I try to stop him from drinking or reason with him, he says that I don't love him anymore. I don't think he really believes he has a problem at all, which is why he can't understand why I get so angry. He's never hit me, but the way I've been abused and degraded is . . . is . . . He just doesn't consider my feelings at all. It's hopeless. I'd leave him, but where can I go?"

Alcoholism is the fourth-largest illness in the world, surpassed only by heart disease, cancer, and mental illness. It shortens the average life span by 11 years. For every healthy person who decides to commit suicide, there are 60 alcoholics. Putting aside for a moment the emotional traumas that it causes, the physical ravages alone are appalling—inflammation and scarring (cirrhosis) of the liver, loss of memory, widespread hemorrhaging, and obesity. Not to mention the defects in babies born to alcoholic mothers—the deformed limbs, distorted faces, and weak hearts.

The opening paragraph of this chapter is a quote from a woman called Deborah. She brought her husband, Jeff, to nutritional counseling in a last bid to save their marriage, and possibly his life. Jeff's decline into alcoholism had followed the classic progression of minute, almost unnoticed stages. He had always enjoyed drinking socially. One reason, he later confessed, was his unease in company—a few drinks relaxed him, allowed him to become friendly and expansive, and he liked thinking of himself as the outgoing center of attention. Gradually, though, he started to drink for the sake of drinking. At work he spent most lunch hours at a bar, usually on his own; at home he went through three bottles of gin a week. If Deborah asked him not to drink so much, he'd use the opportunity to start an argument. It always ended in him angrily walking out of the house. What he refused to admit at the time was that he caused the argument to justify having to go to a bar to cool off.

At work Jeff began to suffer from lapses of memory— forgetting the names of clients, coworkers, and occasionally even his secretary. When he found himself under pressure, he would experience an immediate loss of confidence, start to panic, and find it impossible to stop his hands from shaking—at least, without a drink. He realized later how obvious his drinking must have seemed to his coworkers, but at the time he thought he had everything under wraps. "Once in the elevator someone jokingly warned against putting a match near my mouth for fear of blowing the building up," he recalled. "Well, I turned on him, shouting and ranting, saying that if he had something to say, he should say it, and telling him to mind his own business both at the same time."

Jeff was now drinking continually. He started blacking out and suffering for days on end from nausea and fatigue. He had lost 30 pounds. The flesh on his face sagged, and the tiny cheek capillaries hemorrhaged, giving him a haggard, bruised appearance. He urinated frequently and painfully. His joints ached, and the small of his back felt like a punching bag. Finally, on the recommendation of his doctor, he was admitted to a hospital specializing in alcoholic rehabilitation. In addition to the group therapy and the classes on the damage that alcohol causes, he was made to take a drug that causes violent physical reactions such as stomach cramps, convulsions, and nausea whenever the victim drinks alcohol. A strong aversion to alcohol is meant to result. But within a month of leaving the hospital, Jeff was drinking again.

Finally, on the advice of a friend, Deborah brought Jeff to nutritional counseling. They were shown how amino-based nutritional therapy attacks alcoholism from a radically different angle than conventional treatments. Nutritional counseling looks wholly to inadequate nutrition as the root of the problem, rather than outside events that might be said to have "driven him to drink." Instead of using normal rehabilitative programs, which employ pain, stress, and emotional pressure to force the alcoholic to give up alcohol, amino therapy involves locating the damaged metabolic pathways—those affecting emotional behavior as well as physical well-being—then supplementing and repairing them with an effective blend of amino acids.

Three months after his first consultation, Jeff was a new man. He had stopped drinking completely, and his marriage was on the mend. He had also received the offer of a job from a newly established engineering firm. Each amino constituent of the formulation used to help Jeff was included for the unique way it helped to fight his alcoholism.

We'll look at each of these aminos one by one and then examine the formula Jeff used.

STOPPING THE CRAVING

The first thing to do when treating an alcoholic is to try to stop him from wanting to drink. For this reason, the first amino we'll look at is glutamine. It is one of the most effective supplements available for relieving the alcohol craving. Glutamine is successful because it gently suppresses the mechanism in the brain that causes craving for alcohol. It eradicates the compulsion to drink, which is often such an obstacle to giving it up.

Experts think that it does this by working on the appetite center of the brain's hypothalamus gland. The appetite center's function is to interpret how little or how much food there is in the body. If your body is short of a particular food, the appetite center creates a craving for that one food. When you indulge the craving by eating the food in excess, the nutritional balance is restored.

In the case of alcoholism, many of the people driven to excessive drinking suffer from extremely low blood sugar (hypoglycemia). Responding to this, the appetite center creates an urge to consume foods that raise the levels of sugar circulating in the blood—an urge that, as far as the body is concerned, alcohol meets very successfully. The drawback to this is that, despite the way alcohol initially increases the amount of blood sugar, in the long run it actually causes a drop in these sugar levels. To compensate, the appetite center increases the desire for sugar; the alcoholic drinks more, causing the levels to drop even further, and so on.

Glutamine can break this vicious circle wide open. Remember, glutamine suppresses the brain messages that cause the sugar craving. This allows the blood sugar levels gradually to return to normal and eradicates one of the main reasons for an alcoholic's inability to stop drinking. Glutamine, therefore, is indispensable for the treatment of a variety of alcohol-related disorders.

Glycine is another amino acid that is often used with glutamine to help relieve the cravings of alcoholism and both these aminos are included in the blend at the end of the chapter.

ELIMINATING A CAUSE OF ALCOHOLISM

However, amino acids aren't always so beneficial. For example, excess amounts of the amino leucine are another reason for low blood sugar levels. Nutritionists have found that alcoholism actually increases the levels of leucine in the body, and this is likely to contribute to the victim's hypoglycemia. More important, excess leucine can bring on a variety of mood disorders and physical complaints which only make it harder for the alcoholic to stop drinking. These are caused because leucine allows the kidneys to spill niacin—vitamin B_3—wastefully into the urine.

Niacin is just too important for the body to do without altogether. So when leucine causes a niacin deficiency, the body turns for help to the amino acid tryptophan. One of tryptophan's metabolic pathways produces nicotinanide adenine dinucleotide, a derivative of vitamin B_3. Unfortunately, it takes 60 mg of tryptophan to create 1 mg of B_3, so this process creates a dangerous tryptophan deficiency. Also, tests conducted on the urine of chronically alcoholic patients show that production of the inhibitory neurotransmitter serotonin suffers a drop of 40 percent in the body, which is probably another reason for the mood disorders experienced by alcoholics. We've seen repeatedly how tryptophan, by way of its serotonin-producing pathway, works to relieve stress, anxiety, and depression. Insufficient serotonin prevents the alcoholic from sleeping soundly, and can even lead to aggression and unreasoning anger.

All of these symptoms are typical of chronic alcoholism, and are all caused in a roundabout way by the excess leucine. Reducing the levels of this amino is therefore an ideal way of helping to rehabilitate an alcoholic—raising blood sugar levels, dispelling emotional disorders, and encouraging greater physical well-being.

How do you go about reducing leucine? First, you have to realize that leucine, as well as isoleucine and valine, is a branched-chain amino acid (BCAA). This means that all three must share identically structured transport molecules to move across the intestine wall.

To illustrate this point, think of the BCAAs in the intestines—released from the protein chains and individually waiting for absorption—as a line of travelers standing at a taxi stand. As there are fewer taxis than people, many travelers will have to wait before they can get a ride. In the same way, the branched-chain aminos virtually have to line up to be transported in the bloodstream. Raising the levels of one of these aminos will lead to a depletion of the other two by hogging more of the available transport molecules. Therefore, by taking supplements of isoleucine (one of the competing BCAAs), you can reduce and regulate the amount of leucine that is absorbed. (See the blend at the end of this chapter.)

HELPING YOUR BODY FIGHT THE DISEASE

A lot of the recent research conducted into how and why alcohol affects mood has centered on the way it disrupts the function of brain cells (neurons). Like all cells, the surface membranes of neurons are made of a double skin of fat compounds. Piercing these fatty membranes—jutting out from the cells as well as penetrating them—are many thousands of protein structures that act as receptor sites. These sites are responsible for secreting the neurotransmitting chemicals that convey brain messages across the space between each cell. The uninterrupted passage of impulses along the entire nervous system depends on the efficiency of these receptor sites.

One of the factors that ensures this efficiency is that the fatty cell membranes in which the receptors sit are slightly fluid. This fluidity allows the receptors to move around on the surface. This mobility allows the receptor sites to align themselves precisely. They can, in effect, direct themselves like antennae. This direction-finding ability is important because, in order for a specific brain message to pass from one cell to the next, the structure passing the message on has to locate the similar receptor on the next cell that is designed to receive it.

To put it another way, the thousands of different receptors speak thousands of different languages—one for every sort of message. When a receptor that speaks one language passes a message on, it can only be received by another that speaks the same language. So the slightly fluid surface of the cell lets the receptors quickly and efficiently reposition themselves when searching for another receptor of the same "language."

Alcohol, however, disrupts this process. This is because it is a solvent. The cell wall reacts to it by becoming more fluid, and the balance between mobility and rigidity is tipped over. With nothing to coordinate their messages the receptors are sent haywire—firing off their neurotransmitters without properly aligning themselves, so that their messages are received by receptors that speak different languages.

Not surprisingly, the brain messages become scrambled. Motor commands from the brain to your limbs are garbled, resulting in the loss of balance and coordination typical of drunkenness. Speech centers are affected—you only have to listen to a drunk person talking—the speech is so slurred that his or her tongue sometimes sounds as if it is hamstrung. And contrary to popular belief, it is much harder to fall asleep if you are drunk. Particularly interesting is the way that the receptors that convey pain messages are knocked out. This accounts for the opiatelike feeling of elation that alcohol gives. It also leads to an excess of the excitable neurotransmitter noradrenalin. This is why many people become noisy, agitated, and aggressive when they drink.

Slowly, however, the membranes begin to adapt to the effects of alcohol. To do so, they absorb greater amounts of cholesterol and mineral-based fat compounds. This has the effect of making the cell walls much more rigid. It also accounts for the alcohol tolerance that develops, as ever greater quantities of alcohol are needed to make the cell walls reach that state of fluidity which causes drunkenness. The alcoholic is constantly increasing alcohol consumption simply to reach the same state of euphoria. The resulting depletion of blood sugar only leads him or her to drink more. As we've seen with Jeff, the process quickly spirals out of control.

It also makes it immensely difficult for a chronic alcoholic to stop drinking. By this time, the only way he or she keeps the walls of his or her brain cells in a normal state of fluidity is by drinking excessively. In Malcolm Lowry's extraordinary book about alcoholism, *Under the Volcano*, the drunken hero, Geoffrey Firmin, recognizes "this precarious stage, so arduous to maintain, of being drunk in which he alone was sober." If the alcoholic stops drinking, he is depriving the cell walls of the solvent to dilute them, yet by this time they have adapted themselves to absorb much more hardening material than normal. As a result they become rigid.

This rigidity also causes major problems. First, it leads to a depletion of neurotransmitters—particularly adrenalin. This is a major cause of chronic depression. It leads to fatigue and torpor, a general lack of interest in life that, if continued, soon leads to physical and mental illness. Second, the alcoholic experiences confusion and pain, sometimes even blackouts, as the neurotransmitters that are produced fail to connect with the correct receptors on the now immobile surfaces of the cells. The anxiety, drop in body temperature, and acute shivering of delirium tremens are common results of this.

In these conditions, how could an alcoholic possibly stop drinking? The answer is by using amino acid supplements. Admittedly, the trauma that giving up alcohol causes is intense, but by using amino acids to support the body as alcohol is withdrawn, many of the symptoms can be avoided altogether. To combat the mental fatigue caused by noradrenalin depletion, for example, you can take phenylalanine; tryptophan will replace the lost serotonin; glutamine, as well as regulating the blood sugar levels, works as a brain fuel.

Working together, these aminos help to relieve the mood disorders that are one of the most difficult aspects of alcoholism to treat. But amino acids can also be used to restore fluidity to cell walls. A blend of catabolic aminos (aspartic acid, methionine, and taurine) taken between 4:00 P.M. and 10:00 P.M. breaks down the cholesterol buildup that has taken place in the cell membranes to make them harder. This will help the neurotransmitters to connect effectively and enhance the effects of those mood-improving aminos, while a supplement of carnitine will help carry the excess fats to be burned.

Methionine and taurine are also used to help nurse the liver back to health when the scarring and fat buildup of cirrhosis have taken place.

The effects of alcoholism range throughout the body, and treating it means replacing each and every one of the nutrients that this awful, debilitating disease has stripped away. Only then can an alcoholic reasonably expect to recover. And this is no idle theory. As Jeff and many others have proved, amino acids and their cofactors *do* work.

Here's what Jeff took:

Aminos:
Complete blend
Glutamine
Glycine
Tryptophan
Isoleucine
Phenylalanine
Carnitine
Cofactors:
Vitamin B_3

Vitamin B$_{12}$
Vitamin C
Zinc
Selenium
Catabolic Aminos:
Aspartic acid
Methionine
Taurine
(Best taken between 4:00 P.M. and 10:00 P.M.)

Note: *Please see Chapter 5, "Safety and Precautions," for conditions under which you should not take tryptophan or phenylalanine.*

26

Aid for Anorexia

Anorexia nervosa is a frightening illness. The often extreme physical degeneration of the anorexic and his or her cunning and perverse ways of resisting help are daunting obstacles to overcome. In this illness, as for so many others, amino acid supplements can be an invaluable aid; more and more people affected by anorexia are turning to them for help.

Although some men and many adult women suffer from anorexia, girls in their early to middle teens run the greatest risk of becoming anorexic. In Western Europe and North America, as many as one girl in two hundred is now thought to be suffering from its effects. Often a throwaway comment about the shape of her body is enough to make a girl diet so excessively that she loses control. Or, as she enters puberty, she may experience fear at the powerful changes taking place in her body and try to escape them by starving herself. Because anorexics are often bright, a desire to lose weight can be compounded by parental pressure to excel at school. She will feel that she is being forced into a life over which she has no control. In the face of pressures like this, many girls see the habit of starvation as the only possible way of asserting their individuality. And this habit soon becomes an obsession.

The results are tragic: What little proteins an anorexic does eat are used with their cofactor nutrients simply to keep the body alive. In this life-or-death situation, many nonessential bodily functions are sacrificed. The production of hormones for puberty is halted; menstruation stops. The body quickly reverts to its prepubescent shape, losing a third or more of body weight in the process. The growth into womanhood is effectively arrested. Furthermore, an anorexic's self-perception becomes hideously distorted: As she sinks into her anorexic state, she convinces herself that she is happier and more in control. So, with enormous cunning, she will do all she can to maintain her weight loss.

Free-form amino acids supplements provide a sound nutritional base for recovery from the degeneration caused by the anorexia. By restoring normal functions to the metabolic pathways of the brain, they can alter the anorexics's self-perception, helping her to see her body—often for the first time—as it really is. Most important of all, they can actually make her want to get better.

AMINOCIDE

In previous chapters we've seen how deficiencies of a single nutrient can affect the whole metabolic family. It's rather like flinging a stone into a pool of water; as it sinks it leaves a circular wave that expands to cover the whole surface of the pool. Now, instead of one stone, fling in a hundred all at the same time, and it will give you some idea of the effects of anorexia. For an anorexic simply denies his or her body vital amounts of every nutrient that it needs to live. Accordingly, every single function of the body suffers.

What this all means is that the amino acids that the body must have to function, when eaten at all, are often left to putrefy in the intestines. This in turn produces toxic by-products, which lead to food allergies, vulnerability to infection, fatigue, and a variety of mental and emotional disturbances. Ironically, the metabolic pathways of an anorexic function at such a low ebb that there is often no use for many of the amino acids that do manage, against all the odds, to be absorbed. Instead they might be broken down and released as energy in the form of calories—the thing that anorexics fear most.

When the body's natural balance is so badly disrupted, it is subjected to almost continuous stress—functioning at the second, or resistance, state of the general adaptation syndrome (GAS). To support this stage, the body must have a complete and ample nutritional base. Yet anorexia *destroys* that base.

Sooner or later, an anorexic will succumb to the third stage of GAS—exhaustion. He or she will become even more susceptible to disease (anorexics are notoriously prone to glandular fever) and wounds will take much longer to heal. He or she will start to age prematurely, losing skin tone and hair condition. The ability to concentrate will disappear. He or she will become easily agitated and frightened. All this to a body that, simply to survive, is forced to ravage itself, plundering its own muscles and fat supplies for the amino acids, vitamins, and minerals it needs.

SPECIFICS OF RECOVERY

There is one widespread misconception among therapists and general practitioners treating anorexia, and it highlights the advantages of using free-form amino acids: they believe that reeducating an anorexic to eat, *regardless of what is in his or her diet*, is the most important objective.

It is not. It ignores the anorexic's inability to digest and utilize so much of what is eaten. Often, when the anorexic first starts eating again, his or her stomach and small intestine lack the enzymes needed to break down the food. When this happens, the body simply doesn't get the nutrients that are vital to strengthen the metabolic pathways.

One result will be a painfully slow physical recovery. Another—and for an anorexic far worse—consequence will be a too rapid weight gain. This is because of the damage anorexia causes to the endocrine organs. Many of the hormones these organs secrete, such as thyroxin and growth hormone, are needed by the body to metabolize its food. Without these hormones, food will be converted immediately into calories and will start to accumulate as fat. A runaway weight gain like this is the sort of trauma that causes many a patient to relapse. So we can see that, despite the assertions of many anorexia therapists, specific details of an anorexic's diet are far from unimportant. In rehabilitating an anorexic, they are absolutely essential.

BENEFITS OF AMINO SUPPLEMENTATION

Amino acids help by assisting digestion and the functions of the metabolic pathways so that the patient's physical degeneration is arrested. In a recent study, the amino acid levels of a hundred anorexics were examined. In each case their urinary amino acid profiles showed that they were low in every member of the amino acid family, together with most of the necessary cofactors. Each patient was put on a nutritional first-aid program based on the complete free-form amino blend. In addition, vitamins C, B_6, and E and the minerals calcium, iodine, magnesium, and zinc were also prescribed to encourage efficient metabolization.

Because these amino acids are in their free-form states, anorexics are able to absorb them. They pass straight through the intestinal tract and circulate to wherever they are needed. Arginine and ornithine, for example, generate production of growth hormone. This helps the body use its nutrients properly, metabolizing them into muscle and tissue structure. It also strengthens the immune system.

Phenylalanine, on the other hand, enables the anorexic's body to respond to stress. It also acts as an appetite suppressant, lessening the anorexic's impulse to binge. Carnitine, on the other hand, prevents sudden weight gain by mobilizing the fats in the blood to create energy. And, crucially, cysteine (the most prominent amino acid of the sex hormones FSH and LH) works with calcium to stimulate production of the major female sex hormone, estradiol, enabling growth through puberty to resume. Amino acids also clear toxins from the system, reduce the stress placed on the body by the ravages of anorexia, help make the all-important digestive enzymes, and are generally instrumental in promoting a return to full and balanced health.

The complete amino blend is attractive to anorexics because of its low calorie value. Taking this all-inclusive supplement also spares them the stress of having to spend too much time deciding what to eat. Because of their high nutritional value, they can be taken initially with smaller amounts of food than would otherwise be healthy, easing the anorexic gently into the habit of eating solid food.

THE SELF-DECEPTION

Giving the anorexic physical support is important, but there is much more to the treatment than this. The disastrous effects on the body are only symptoms of the true nature of anorexia: the anorexic's distorted view of the internal and external world. When an anorexic looks in a mirror, face-to-face with the emaciated shadow of what she once was, all she sees is obesity. Stepping on a scale and finding she has gained a few ounces, all she feels is self-hatred. When confronted with the increasing alarm of her friends and relations, she diverts their attention away from herself, playing one person off against another, putting herself across as the wronged and defenseless party to avoid facing her problem. Every aspect of her life becomes deadened by her morbid self-obsession.

Clearly, anorexia stems from severe disturbances of the body image—disturbances that are created in the mind. Here, too, amino acids can prove immensely helpful. Amino acid supplements strengthen the metabolic pathways of the brain, helping alter mood, mental functioning, and behavior.

The Perception Aminos

A major cause of the mental and emotional disturbances of anorexia is thought to lie with imbalances in the brain's neurotransmitters. Studies show that when serotonin levels are low, people behave abnormally, often overreacting to stimuli. Because of this, serotonin has been found effective in combat'ng a variety of compulsive disorders, particularly the obsessive behavior of anorexia. The precursor of serotonin is the amino acid tryptophan, so additional doses of tryptophan are often prescribed on top of amounts contained in the full blend. Another substance found to be effective in helping the brain functions of anorexics is glutamine.

Finally, we come to the amino acid asparagine. Along with glutamic acid, it is the most commonly found amino in the brain. As it is present in such high quantities, researchers think it must play a major role in maintaining optimum brain function, helping to regulate the metabolism of the brain and cells of the nervous system. In fact, people with emotional and behavioral problems almost invariably suffer from low levels of asparagine. In a recent test, 150 out of 152 patients experiencing severe emotional and behavioral disorders were found to have levels of asparagine well below the norm. When they took it as a supplement, all the patients reported a growth in self-confidence and an increased desire to face the problems of their lives head on. You'll find tryptophan, asparagine, and their cofactors listed in the recovery formula at the end of the chapter.

HAPPY ENDINGS

More and more people whose lives have been ruined by anorexia are turning to amino acids for help. Mary was a 29-year-old nurse who had waged an on-and-off battle with anorexia since her midteens. Over a period of about 12 years, she had visited six psychiatrists. After each course of treatment she staged a recovery, only to relapse back into her anorexic obsession after two months or so. She had never menstruated fully. Despite her starved appearance, looking years beyond her age, she denied that she felt particularly ill. She was immediately put on the full amino blend, together with additional tryptophan and glutamine— agreeing to take them only because of their low calorie values.

After only a few days of taking the supplements, the change in her attitude was astonishing: "I looked in the mirror and was stunned to see how horribly thin I was. My perceptions had changed overnight. All that time when I was convinced of my obesity, I was actually little more than a scarecrow." With a newfound sense of lucidity giving her the determination to recover, she started a whole-food diet supplemented by free-form amino acids and their cofactors. Within three months, she was healthier than she'd been in her life.

Lois was a 41-year-old woman who had been made to seek help by her worried son. She denied that there was anything seriously wrong with her, and she was noncommittal and secretive when questioned about her anorexia. After taking the complete blend for less than a week, she confessed that she was bulimic (making herself vomit after she ate) as well as anorexic, and had been so for almost 20 years. In the last five years, the illness had progressively worsened. She had lost her job, and her husband had left her. She felt constantly on the verge of a nervous breakdown and suffered from insomnia, lack of concentration, and extreme fatigue.

As well as the full amino blend, she was given extra asparagine, tryptophan, and glutamine, together with their cofactors. Within a short while, she had staged a remarkable recovery. She felt strong and full of physical energy. Furthermore, she was mentally composed and alert—a stark contrast to her former unfocused and hyperactive state of mind (so characteristic of anorexia). She met her second husband soon after on a skiing holiday in Italy.

As encouraging as these examples are, the disturbing fact

is that these women, both well into adulthood, had been
anorexic since their teens. They had repeatedly sought help
and been treated by psychiatrists whose attitude seemed to
be, "get them used to eating, and the battle is won." In
many less severe cases, this approach probably works, but
it's a desperately hit-or-miss affair. Most anorexics who do
recover admit to "constantly having to look over my
shoulder, knowing that the specter of anorexia is still
there." Not surprisingly, many suffer a relapse. Getting the
anorexic to start eating and then simply hoping for the best
is not the answer, as Mary and Lois will testify. Sadly, there
seems to be a gulf between the therapist's aims—which are
to help anorexics to recover—and their methods, which are
to feed them with literally anything that comes to hand.

Free-form amino acids can bridge that gulf. They supply
in a concentrated and balanced form all the nutrients an
anorexic needs to recover physiologically. At the same time
they help the brain to work properly. Striking at the very
heart of the illness, they can restore a patient's balance,
perception, and lucidity.

This formula includes all of the nutrients mentioned in
this chapter to aid in the anorexic's recovery:

Aminos:
Complete blend
Tryptophan
Glutamine
Arginine
Asparagine
Cofactors:
Vitamin C
Vitamin B$_6$
Vitamin E
Calcium
Iodine
Magnesium
Zinc

Note: *Please see Chapter 5, "Safety and Precautions," before
taking aminos.*

Final Words

This book has given you a great deal of information on the nutritional value of free-form amino acids and how you can use them to their best advantage. This has often meant exploring the workings of the body's metabolic pathways. Perhaps at times this maze of interlocking biochemical routes has seemed confusing. If so, just remember that a maze can confuse only as long as you don't know your way around it. Once you have a map, you can easily and swiftly reach your destination.

That's where this book comes in. *The Amino Revolution* is something of a treasure map: It helps you find your way around the metabolic pathways. This means knowing which amino supplements to use so that each metabolic pathway can function at peak performance.

The treasures that await you? Increased mental, emotional, and physical well-being through the health-enhancing potential of free-form amino acids.

Just follow the map.

References

Chapter 1
Ajinomoto Co., *Amino Acids* (Part 3), Tokyo, 1980.
Chaitow, L., *Amino Acids in Therapy*, Thorsons, New York, 1985.
Greerstein, J. and Winitz, M., *Chemistry of Amino Acids*, Wiley, New York, 1931.
Guyton, A., *Textbook of Medical Physiology*, 5th edition, Saunder, 1976.
Meister, A., *Biochemistry of Amino Acids*, 2nd edition, Academic Press, New York, 1965.
Rose, S., *The Chemistry of Life*, Pelican, London, 1985.

Chapter 2
Bremer, H., and others, *Disturbances of Amino Acid Metabolism: Clinical Chemistry and Diagnosis*, Urban and Schwarzenberg, Baltimore, 1981.
Lehninger, A., *Biochemistry: The Molecular Basis of Cell Structure and Function*, Worth Publishers, New York, 1970.

McGilvery, R., *Biochemistry: A Functional Approach*, Saunders, London, 1970.

Chapter 3
Bender, D., *Amino Acid Metabolism*, Wiley, 1985.
Colgen, M., *Your Personal Vitamin Profile*, Quill, New York, 1982.
Devlin, T., *Textbook of Biochemistry with Clinical Applications*, Wiley, 1982.
Jo-Mar Laboratories, "Introduction to the Amazing Amino Acids with Their Strange-Sounding Names," Booklet 1, Los Gatos, California, 1981.
Munro, H., and Crim, M., "The Proteins and Amino Acids," in *Modern Nutrition in Health and Disease*, edited by Goodhart and Shils, 5th edition, 1978.

Chapter 5
"Adaptive Responses of Amino Acid Degrading Enzymes to Variations of Amino Acid and Protein Intake," *Nutritional Reviews*, Nov. 1976.
Filer, L. J., and others, "Plasma Amino-Grams in Infants and Adults Fed an Identical High Protein Meal," *Fed Prog.* 36, 1977, 1181.
Forbes, A., "Regulation of Oral Amino Acid Preparations," *Clinical Nutritional Update*, Amer. Medic. Assoc., Chicago, 1977.
Harper, A. E., and others, "Effects of Ingestion of Disproportionate Amounts of Amino Acids," *Physiol. Rev.* 50, 1970, 428.
Snyderman, S., "Levels of the Anomalies of Amino Acid Metabolism," *Amino Acids Clinical Nutrition Update American Medical Association*, Chicago, 1977, 159–166.
Stegink, L. D., "Absorption, Utilization and Safety of Aspartic Acid," *J. Toxicol, and Environ. Health*, 2, 1976, 215.

Chapter 6
Meiss, D., and others, "Amino Acid Analysis: An Important Nutritional and Clinical Evaluation Tool," *Nutr. Perspectives*, 6 (2) 1983, 19–24.

Rattenbury, J., *Amino Acid Analysis*, Halsted Press, 1981.

Salaman, M., "Amino Acid Testing," *Let's Live*, Aug. 1984, 82–83.

Stryer, L., *Biochemistry*, Freeman Co., San Francisco, 1975.

Chapter 7

Bland, J., *Medical Applications of Clinical Nutrition*, Keats, 1983.

Lessor, M., *Nutrition and Vitamin Therapy*, Grove Press, New York, 1980.

Chapter 9

Barbul and others, "Thymotropic Actions of Arginine, Ornithine and Growth Hormone," *Fed. Proc.*, 1978, 282.

Butler, R., and others, "The Effects of Preloads of Amino Acids on Short-Term Satiety," *American Journal of Clinical Nutrition*, Oct. 1982, 2045–47.

Fox, A., *The Beverly Hills Medical Diet*, Bantam Books, 1981.

Isidori and others, "A Study of Growth Hormone Release in Man After Oral Administration of Amino Acids," *Curr. Med. Res. Opi.*, 475–81.

Kenton, L., *Biogenic Diet*, Century, 1986.

Koppf and others, "Plasma Growth Hormone Response to Intravenous Administration of Amino Acids," *J. Clin. Endocr.*, 25, 1985, 1140–44.

McDougall, J., and McDougall, M., *The McDougall Plan*, New Century Publishers, 1985.

Merinee and others, "Arginine-Initiated Release of Human Growth Hormone," *New Engl. J. Med.*, 183(26), 1969, 1425–29.

Newbold, H., *Dr. Newbold's Revolutionary New Discoveries About Weight Loss*, Rawson Assoc., 1977.

Passwater, R., *Supernutrition for a Healthy Heart*, Dial Press, 1977.

Pearson and Shaw, *The Life Extension Weight Loss Program*, Doubleday, 1986.

Scriver, C., and Rosenbury, L., *Amino Acid Metabolism and Its Disorders*, Saunders, Philadelphia, 1973.

Wade, C., *The New Enzyme Catalyst Diet*, Parker Publishing, 1976.

Williams, R., *Nutrition Against Disease*, Bantam Books, 1981.

Chapter 10

Ader, R. (ed.), *Psychoneuroimmunology*, Academic Press, New York, 1981.

Barchas, J., and others, "Behavioral Neurochemistry: Neuroregulators and Behavioral States," *Science 200*, May 26, 1976, 964–73.

Bender, D., *Amino Acid Metabolism*, Wiley, 1985.

Bland, J., *Medical Applications of Clinical Nutrition*, Keats, 1983.

Butter, C., *Neuropsychology: The Study of Brain and Behavior*, Brooks Cole, 1969.

Cooper, J., and others, *The Biochemical Basis of Neuropharmacology*, Oxford Press, 1978.

Curson, G. (ed.), *The Biochemistry of Psychiatric Disturbances*, Wiley, 1980.

DeFeudis, "Amino Acids as Central Neurotransmitters," *Ann. Res. Pharmacol.*, 15, 1975, 105–127.

Fernstrom, J., "Effects of Precursors on Brain Neurotransmitter Synthesis and Brain Functions," *Diabetologia*, 1981, 20:281–89.

Frank, B., *Dr. Frank's No-Aging Diet*, Dial Press, 1978.

Green, A., and Costain, D., *Pharmacology and Biochemistry of Psychiatric Disorders*, Wiley, 1981.

Hawkins, D., and Pauling, L., *Orthomolecular Psychiatry*, Freeman, San Francisco, 1973.

Hoffa, A., "Mega Amino Acid Therapy," *Ortho. Psych.*, Vol. 9, 1983, 2–5.

Iverson, L., and others, *Handbook of Psychopharmacology*, Plenum Press, 1978.

Longo, V. F., *Neuropharmacology and Behavior*, Freeman, 1972.

Passwater, R., "Notes on Stress, Heart Attacks and Problems of the Mind," *Health Quarterly Journal*, Vol. 5, Nov.–Dec. 1980.

Pfeiffer, C., *Mental and Elemental Nutrients*, Keats, 1975.

Quastel, J., "The Role of Amino Acids in the Brain," essays in *Medical Biochemistry*, Vol. 4, London, 1979.

Reichelt and Kyamme, "Acetylated and Peptide-Bound Glutamate and Aspartate in the Brain," *Journal of Neurochemistry*, 14, 1967, 987.

Seiden, L., and Dykstra, L., *Psychopharmacology: A Biochemical and Behavioral Approach*, Van Nostrand, 1977.

Watson, G., *Nutrition and Your Mind: The Psychochemical Response*, Harper and Row, London, 1972.

Chapter 11

Barbul and others, "Arginine, a Thymotropic and Wound-Healing Promoting Agent," *Surgical Forum*, 28: 1977, 101–03.

Beisel, W. R., "Malnutrition as a Consequence of Stress," in *Malnutrition in the Immune Responses*, Suskind (ed.). Raven Press, New York, 1977.

Blackburn and others, "Branched Chained Amino Acids Administration and Metabolism During Starvation, Injury and Infection," *Surgery* 86, 1979, 307–15.

Border and others, "Multiple Systems Organ Failure: Muscle Fuel Deficit with Visceral Protein Malnutrition," *Surgery* 56, 1976, 1147–50.

Cerra and others, "Septic Autocannibalism: a Failure of Exogeneous Nutritional Support," *Ann. Surgery*, 1980.

Cerra, F., and others, "Branched Chains Support Postoperative Protein Synthesis," *Surgery* 92, 1982, 192–9.

Cuthbertson, D., and others, "Metabolism During the Post Injury Period," *Adv. Cln. Chem.*, 1969, 12211–55.

Waterlow, J., and others, "The Measurement of Rates of Protein Turnover, Synthesis and Breakdown in Man and the Effects of Nutritional Status and Surgical Injury," *American Journal of Nutrition* 30, 1977, 1933–39.

Chapter 12

Cheraskin & Ringsdorf, *Psychodietetics*, Bantam, New York, 1976.

Ellis, J., and others, "Flight-Induced Changes in Human Amino Acid Excretion," *Aviation, Space and Environment Med.* 1–8, Jan. 1976.

Growdon, J. H., & Wurtman, R., "Dietary Influences on the Synthesis of Neurotransmitters in the Brain," *Nutr. Rev.* 37, 1979, 129–36.

Hale, H., and others, "Human Amino Acid Excretion Patterns During and Following Prolonged Multistressor Tests," *Aviation, Space and Environmental Med.*, Feb. 1975, 173–78.

Hawkins, P., and others, "Amino Acid Supply to Individual Cerebral Structures in Awake and Anesthetized Rats," *Amer. Physiol. Soc.*, E1–11, 1982.

Hoffer, *Orthomolecular Nutrition,*" Keats, Connecticut, 1978.

Chapter 13

Barchas, J., and others, "Behavioral Neurochemistry, Neuroregulators and Behavioral States," *Science* 200, May 26, 1978, 964–73.

Cherkin, A. & Van Harreveld, A., "L-Proline and Related Compounds: Correlation of Structure Amnesic Potency and Anti-Spreading Depression Potency," *Brain Research* 156, 1978, 265–73.

Geldenberg, A., and others, "Tyrosine for Treatment of Depression," *Am. J. of Psychiatry*, 137, 1980, 622–32.

Goldberg, I., "L-Tyrosine in Depression," *Lancet* 2, 1980, 364.

Hawkins, D., & Pauling, L., *Orthomolecular Psychiatry*, Freeman, San Francisco, 1973.

Pearson, D., & Shaw, S., *Life Extension*, Warner, 1982.

Pearson, D., & Shaw, S., *The Life Extension Companion*, Warner, 1984.

Rose, W., and others, "The Amino Acid Requirements of Man. The Phenyalanine Requirement," *J. Biol. Chem.*, 213, 1955, 913–22.

Chapter 14

Scriver, C., & Rosenberg, L., *Amino Acid Metabolism and Its Disorders*, W. B. Saunders, 1973.

Stanbury, J., and others, *The Metabolic Basis of Inherited Disease*, McGraw-Hill, 1978.
Williams, R., *Nutrition Against Disease*, Bantam Books, 1981.

Chapter 15
Critslis, A. N. et. al., "Arginine Inhibits a Viral Tumor," (abstract), *Fed. Proc.* 36:1163, 1977.
Barbul, A., et al., "Arginine: A Thymotropic and Wound-Healing Promoting Agent," *Surgical Forum* 28: 101–103, 1977.
Milner, J. A., and Stepanovich, L. V., "Inhibitory Effect of Dietary Arginine on Growth of Ehrlich Ascites Tumor Cells in Mice," *J. Nutr.* 109, 489, 1979.
Rettura et al., "Supplemental Arginine Increases Thymic Cellularity in Normal and Murine Sarcoma Virus-Innoculated Mice and Increases the Resistance to Murine Sarcoma Virus Tumor," *J. Parent. Enteral Nutr.* 3, 409, 1979.

Chapter 16
Bland, J., *Medical Applications of Clinical Nutrition*, Keats, 1983.
Journal of American Medical Association, Dec. 15, 1978, 2712–14.
Pearson and Shaw, *Life Extension*, Warner, 1982.
"Proteins,"*Nutrition Reports International*, Sept. 1983, 497–507.
Sanchez, A., and others, "Plasma Amino Acids in Humans."
Sved, A., and others, "Studies on the Antihypertensive Action of L-tryptophan," *J. of Pharm. and Exp. Therapeutic*, Vol. 221, 1982, 329–33.

Chapter 17
"The Importance of Gastrointestinal pH Balance," *Bulletin of Heidelberg International*, Norcross, GA 30092.

246 THE AMINO REVOLUTION

Chapter 18

Levine, S., and Kidd, P., *Antioxidant Adaptation*, Allergy Research Group, San Leandro, CA, 1985.

Phillpot, W., & Kalita, D., *Brain Allergies*, Keats, 1981.

Phillpot, W., & Kalita, D., *Victory over Diabetes*, Keats, 1983.

Chapter 19

Lessor, M., *Nutrition and Vitamin Therapy*, Grove Press, New York, 1980.

Mann, T., *The Biochemistry of Semen and the Male Reproductive Tract*, Wiley, 1964.

Pfeiffer, C., *Mental and Elemental Nutrients*, Keats, 1975.

Pryor, J., and others, "Controlled Clinical Trial of Arginine for Infertile Men with Oligozoospermin," *Br. T. Urol. 50(1), Feb. 1978, 47–50.*

Chapter 20

Griffith, R., and others, "A Multicentered Study of Lysine Therapy in Herpes Simplex Infection," *Dermatologica* 156(5), 1978, 256–67.

Milman, N., and others, "Lysine Prophylaxis in Recurrent Herpes Simplex Labialic," *Acta Dorm Venereol*, (Stockh) 60, 1980, 85–87.

Sanchez, A., and others, "Plasma Amino Acids in Human Fed Plant Proteins," *Nutritional Reports International*, Sept. 1983, 497–507.

Chapter 21

Blackburn and others, *Amino Acids*, John Wright, 1983.

Davidson, A., and others, "Brain Decarboxylase Activities as Indices of Pathological Change in Senile Dementia," *Lancet*, 1974, 1247.

Hoffer, A., and Walker, M., *Nutrients to Age Without Senility*, Keats, 1980.

Kenton, L., *Ageless Aging*, Century, 1985.

Levine, S., and Kidd, P., *Antioxidant Adaptation*, Allergy Research Group, San Leandro, CA, 1985.

Lundholm, K., "Aging Amino Acid and Protein Metabolism."

Wade, C., *Miracle Protein*, Parker Publishing, New York, 1975.

Chapter 22

Bondy, P., and Rosenberg, L., *Metabolic Control and Disease*, 8th ed., Saunders, Philadelphia, 1980.

Stryer, L., *Biochemistry*, S. H. Freeman, San Francisco, 1975.

Chapter 23

Sprince, H., and others, "Comparison of Protection by L-Ascorbic Acid, L-Cysteine, and Adrenergic-Blocking Agents Against Acetaldehyde, Acrolein, and Formaldehyde Toxicity, Implications in Smoking," *Agents and Actions* 9, 1979, 407.

Chapter 24

Ikeda, H., "Effects of Taurine on Alcohol Withdrawal," *Lancet*, Sept. 1977, 509.

Lowry, M., *Under the Volcano*, Penguin, London, 1983.

Morgan, M., and others, "Ratio of Plasma Amino-n-Butyric Acid to Leucine as an Empirical Marker of Alcoholism," *Science*, Sept. 16, 1977, 1183–85.

Ravel, J., and others, "Reversal of Alcohol Toxicity by Glutamine," *Journ. Biol. Chem.*, Vol. 214, 1955, 497–501.

Rogers, L., "Some Biological Effects of Glutamine," *Am. Chem. Soc.*, Houston, Dec. 1955.

Rogers, L., and Pelton, "Glutamine in the Treatment of Alcoholism," *Quarterly Jour. of Studies on Alcohol*, Vol. 18, No., 4, 1957.

Trunnel, J., and Wheeler, J., "Preliminary Report on Experiments with Orally Administered Glutamine Treatment in Treatment of Alcoholics," *Am. Chem. Soc.*, Dec. 1955.

Williams, R., *Alcoholism: The Nutritional Approach*, Univ. of Texas, 1959.

Chapter 25

Newbold, H., *Mega-Nutrients for Your Nerves*, Peter Wyden Press, New York, 1975.

Quastel, J., "The Role of Amino Acids in the Brain," essays in *Medical Biochemistry*, Vol. 4, Great Britain, 1979, 1-48.

Reinis, S., and Goldman, J., *The Chemistry of Behavior*, Plenum Press, New York, 1982.

Wurtman, R., "Nutrients That Modify Brain Function," *Scientific Amer.*, April 1982.

Chapter 26

Bender, D., *Amino Acid Metabolism*, 2nd edition, Wiley, 1985.

Blackburn and others (eds.), *Amino Acid Metabolism and Medical Applications*, John Wright, 1983.

Cunningham-Rundles, S., "Effects of Nutritional Status on Immunological Function," *Amer. Jour. of Clin. Nutr.*, May 1982, 1202-10.

Wright, J., and Gaby, A., "Clinical Applications of Nutritional Biochemistry," Seminar, San Francisco, 1983.